Color Atlas of
Meat and Poultry Inspection

Geoffrey S. Wiggins
MRCVS, Veterinary Officer, City
of London

Andrew Wilson
MRCVS, DVSM, Chief Veterinary
Officer, City of Birmingham

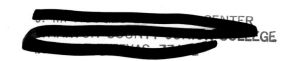

VNR VAN NOSTRAND REINHOLD COMPANY
NEW YORK   CINCINNATI   ATLANTA   DALLAS   SAN FRANCISCO

Acknowledgements

We are grateful to the Ministry of Agriculture, Fisheries and Food for supplying the following illustrations which are Crown Copyright, and for the kind permission of the Controller of HMSO, to include them: Nos. 30, 38, 49, 109, 110, 111, 112, 113, 114, 115, 116, 117, 118, 184, 232, 233, 234, 285, 307, 308, 314 and 319.

Mr David Howie, MRCVS, DVSM, was also kind enough to supply the following: Nos. 4, 51, 67, 77, 85, 100, 120, 121, 125, 161, 173, 175, 194, 197, 221, 230, 231, 237, 238 and 262, and the Royal Veterinary College, No. 245.

We are also very grateful to Mr J. Baker, FAPHI, FRSH, for his very valuable help with the Poultry section.

We should also like to thank the publishers for help and advice in producing the book, and Miss C. Lovett for her technical assistance.

Introduction

This atlas is the first to deal with meat and poultry inspection in full color, and the first to illustrate comprehensively a wide range of conditions, making them easily recognizable when they arise in the course of inspection. It is therefore an invaluable aid to inspectors wishing to keep up to date with standards of meat and poultry inspection. This is specially true now that some countries have already adopted rigorous and uniform standards.

The book is in two sections: Meat Inspection and Poultry Inspection. The photographs of the diseases and conditions have been arranged alphabetically, using the most common names and not necessarily the scientific ones, although the latter are also given in the text and in the index. To help the reader find a particular condition, the list of contents has been arranged under the type of animal and its various parts – for example, **SHEEP**, kidney, liver, and so on.

Almost all the illustrations are of animals which have been slaughtered and bled. Photographs of those which have died, and therefore not bled, are clearly indicated as such in the text.

Our aim has been to produce a comprehensive selection of conditions which the inspector is likely to see in the slaughterhouse. Obviously it would be almost impossible to include all conditions, but the adage 'common things are common' holds good, and it is on such common things that we have concentrated, although there are also photographs of other conditions which are rare but nevertheless important.

The appearance of any particular condition changes constantly during the course of the disease. These pictures show a pathological process at a particular stage in its development but we have selected those appearances that are as near 'typical' as possible. The text has been kept deliberately short as most of the illustrations are self-explanatory.

The book is meant as a guide to all those involved in the field of meat or poultry inspection and should be specially useful to veterinary surgeons, environmental health officers, authorised meat inspectors and students of those professions. If, apart from instruction, it can be used to assist or endorse a judgment, the authors will have achieved their object.

Contents

All numbers in bold type refer to illustrations

Meat

ABSCESS

1. BOVINE LIVER. The commonest cause is *Fusiformis necrophorus*. The abscesses can become very large, often with adhesions to the other viscera and the parietal peritoneum.

2. PIG. *Corynebacterium pyogenes* is commonly associated with abscesses in pigs. The pus is often lime green in colour.

3. PIG. Note that the pus is becoming inspissated and that a fibrous capsule has formed (*arrow*).

4. PIG KIDNEY SUBSTANCE. Note that the rest of the kidney is normal. Occasionally organs will completely reject heavily encapsulated abscesses.

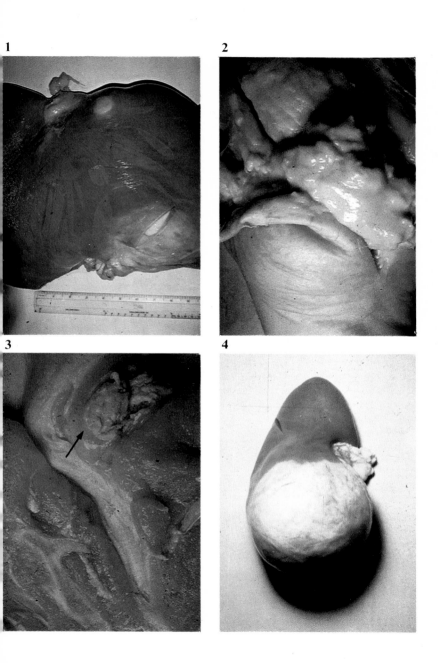

1

2

3

4

ABSCESS, cont.

5. PIG VERTEBRAE. These are sequelae of a damaged (bitten) tail. See **174**.

6. PIG SPINAL CORD. Spinal and pelvic abscesses often result from bitten tails. This pig was partially paralysed in the hind legs.

7. SHEEP NECK. This is an abscess probably caused by a hypodermic injection. Note the wool contained in the abscess. Strands of wool were possibly forced into the tissues by the hypodermic needle and, still attached, had continued to grow.

8. SHEEP ELBOW. A likely cause would be organisms entering via the skin.

9. SHEEP. This is a pyaemic spread from abscess on elbow (see **8**). Note the abscesses in the lung, heart, liver and kidneys. Evidence of lung worm (*Muellerius capillaris*) infestation can also be seen.

10. PIG LUNGS. Pyaemic spread.

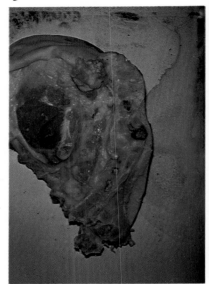

8

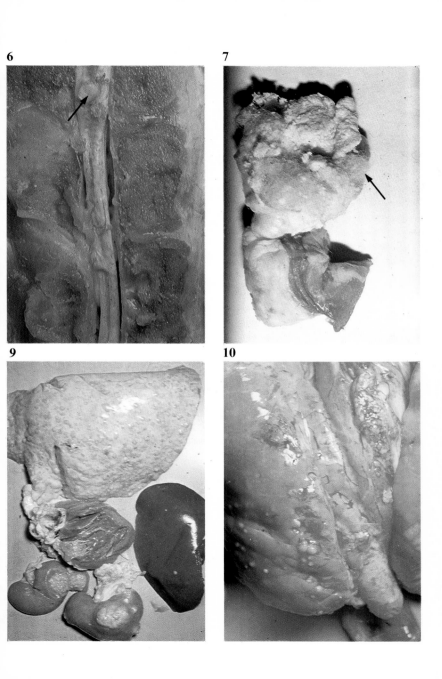

ABSCESS, cont.

11. CALF KIDNEY. Pyaemic spread from an umbilical pyaemia (see **273** and **274**).

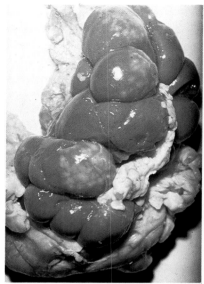

12. BOVINE LIVER. Pyaemic spread. Note also the yellow colour of the liver due to fatty infiltration (see **102**).

ACTINOBACILLOSIS

13. BOVINE TONGUE ('WOODEN TONGUE'). The causal organism is *Actinobacillus lignièresi*. Note that the lesions generally appear on the unprotected side of the tongue. Typical nodules are at A in the substance and at B where they appear as nodular swellings under the mucous membrane.

14. BOVINE LYMPH NODES. Note on the cut surface how the lesions protrude. In some of the nodules there are specks of pus (*arrow*). This is bright yellow in appearance and is granular.

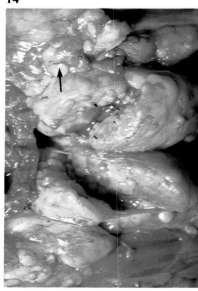

15. BOVINE LYMPH NODE. This is an older lesion than **14**. Note the white fibrous tissue surrounding the nodules (*arrow*). The formation of this fibrous tissue is very characteristic of actinobacillosis.

16. BOVINE SOFT AND HARD PALATES. Note the shallow ulcers indicated by the two arrows. These are lesions which can often be overlooked. Note also the black pigmentation which commonly occurs in the bovine mouth.

12

13

15

16

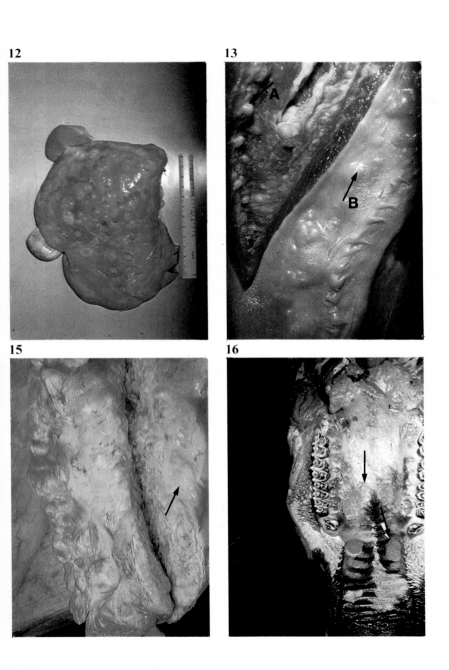

ACTINOBACILLOSIS, cont.

17. BOVINE MASSETER MUSCLE. The typical nodules are plainly visible.

18. BOVINE NECK MUSCLE. Note that the nodules run in lines (*arrow*), probably in the lymphatic vessels.

19. BOVINE OESOPHAGUS. The oesophageal wall is grossly thickened (*arrow*) due to numerous nodules.

20. BOVINE OESOPHAGUS (CLOSE-UP). The oesophageal wall is grossly thickened with closely packed nodules which protrude from the cut surface.

21. BOVINE LUNG. Infection is probably by inhalation.

22. BOVINE LIVER. The protruding nodules on the cut surface are interspersed with the typical white fibrous tissue. Compare with tuberculosis of bovine liver (**252**). Infection is via the blood stream or spread from an adjacent infected organ, e.g. the reticulum.

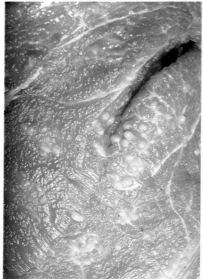

17

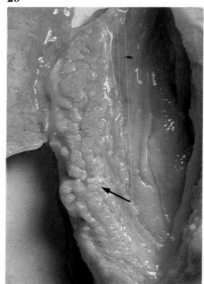

20

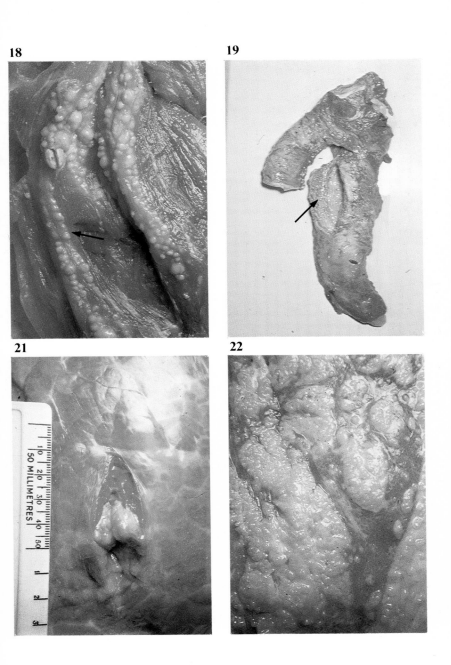

ACTINOBACILLOSIS, cont.

23. BOVINE RETICULUM, WITH NORMAL RETICULUM ON THE LEFT. The wall of the affected reticulum is grossly thickened (A) with damaged mucous membrane (B).

24. BOVINE PERITONEUM. This shows the typical nodules. There are also lesions in the kidney. The picture demonstrates how the condition could be confused with tuberculosis (**250**).

ACTINOMYCOSIS

25. BOVINE JAW, MANDIBLE ('LUMPY JAW'). This causal organism is *Actinomyces bovis*. This is a fairly early lesion showing an abscess with extensive fibrous encapsulation. This leads to a rarefying osteitis and granuloma as is seen in **26** and **27**.

26. BOVINE JAW. The lesion has been sawn through to show the deep seated abscesses and fistulae.

27. BOVINE MANDIBLE ('LUMPY JAW'). The typical swelling is shown (*arrow*). As the inner bone disintegrates new bone is laid down on the outside to maintain the tensile strength.

23

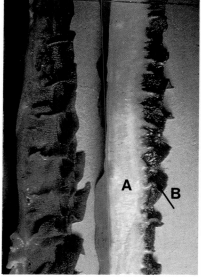

26

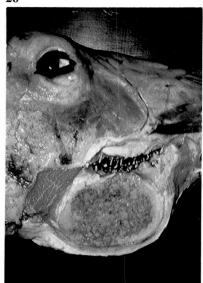

24

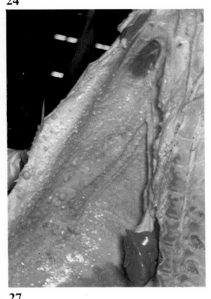

25

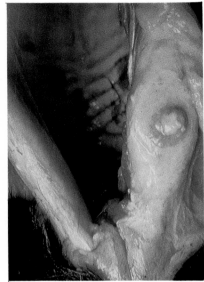

27

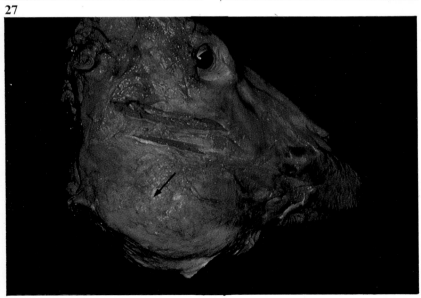

ACTINOMYCOSIS, cont.

28. SOW MAMMARY GLANDS. The lesions are similar to those in bovine actinobacillosis. Note the deep seated nodules and the dense fibrous tissue (*arrow*).

ANTHRACOSIS (AND TUBERCULOSIS)

29. BOVINE BRONCHIAL LYMPH NODES. The black areas of anthracosis, due to the inhalation of carbon particles or coal dust, are scattered throughout the substance.

ANTHRAX

30. BOVINE BLOOD. The causal organism is *Bacillus anthracis*. This is a large rod shaped bacillus with square cut ends. The organism is capsulated in body fluids. This blood smear has been stained with MacFadyean's methylene blue. The bacilli are stained blue and the capsular material violet.

ARTHRITIS

31. SHEEP STIFLE JOINT. The condition is usually reflected in the iliac lymph nodes. When detecting enlarged joints it is helpful to be able to compare both sides of a carcase.

32. CALF STIFLE JOINT, SEPTIC ARTHRITIS ('JOINT ILL'). Note the enlarged internal iliac lymph node (*arrow*). This is a common sequela of umbilical pyaemia ('navel ill'). See **273** and **274**.

28

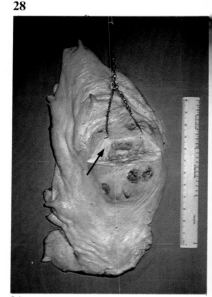

31

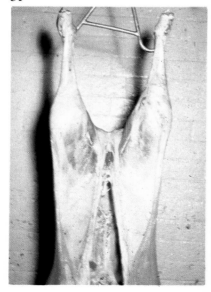

29

30

32

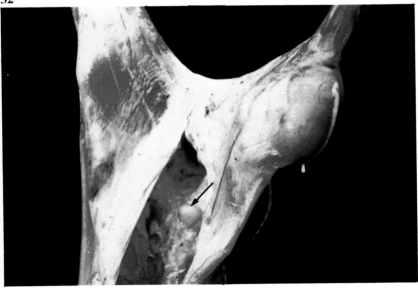

ARTHRITIS, cont.
33. SHEEP HOCK JOINT.

ASCARIASIS
34. PIG LIVER ('MILK SPOT'). This shows damage to the liver caused by the ascaris larvae.

35. PIG LIVER ('MILK SPOT'). Milk spot liver can also be caused occasionally by other conditions such as avian tuberculosis.

ASCARIS SUUM (A. LUMBRICOIDES)
36. EX. INTESTINE PIG.

ATELECTASIS
37. BOVINE FOETAL LUNGS. The lungs are liver like in appearance.

33

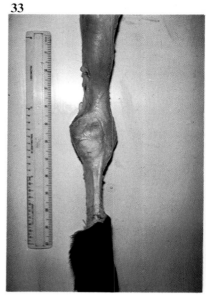

36

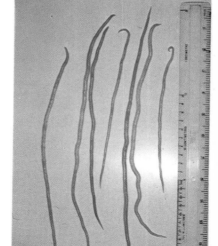

34

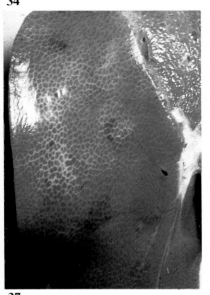

35

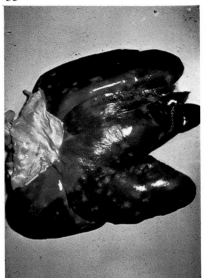

37

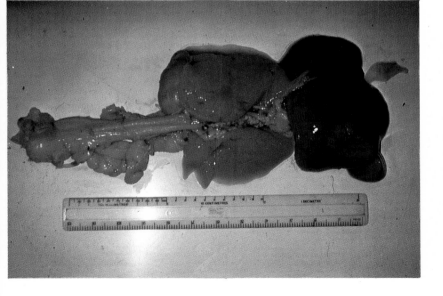

ATROPHIC RHINITIS
38. PIG. The face is distorted.

39. PIG. Note the distortion of the nasal septum.

'BACK BLEEDING' ('OVERSTICKING')
40. PIG. Note the blood in the thoracic cavity (A) and behind the sternum and ribs (B).

BLACKQUARTER (BLACKLEG, QUARTER-EVIL)
41. BOVINE MUSCLE. The causal organism is usually *Clostridium chauvoei*. The disease, sometimes called pseudoanthrax, runs a rapid course, death being brought about by acute toxaemia.

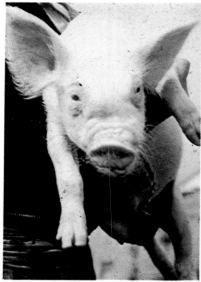

38

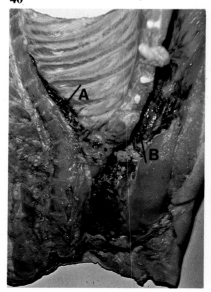

40

39

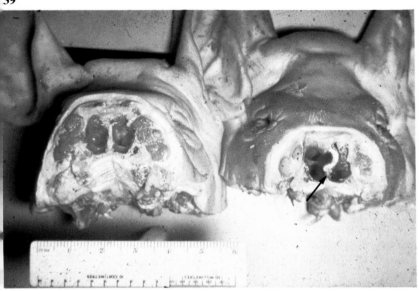

41

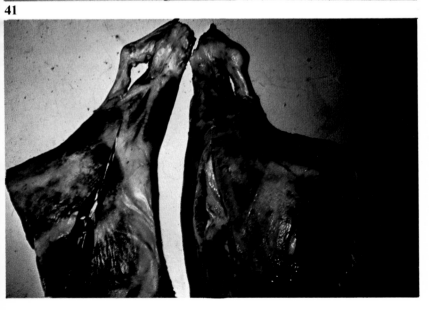

BLACKQUARTER, cont.

42. BOVINE MUSCLE. This is a close-up of **41** showing acute inflammation (A), a gangrenous area (B) and gas spaces (C).

'BLACKSPOT' MOULD (*CLADOSPORIUM HERBARUM*)

43. SHEEP. This is an imported frozen carcase.

'BLACKSPOT' MOULD AND 'WHITESPOT' (*SPOROTRICHON CARNIS*)

44. SHEEP. The pleura and peritoneum are affected. This is also an imported frozen carcase.

BLOOD SPLASHING

45. PIG LUNG. The haemorrhages occur during slaughter. They are most common when electrical stunning is used, particularly when there is a delay in 'sticking'.

46. BOVINE MUSCLE.

47. LAMB INTESTINES AND MESENTERY. The condition is commoner in young animals, probably because of the fragility of the capillary walls.

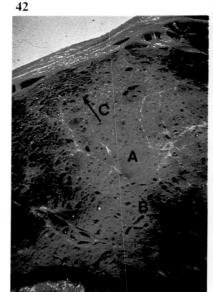

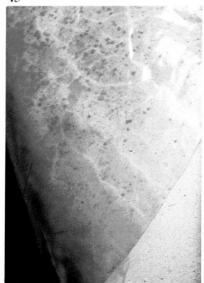

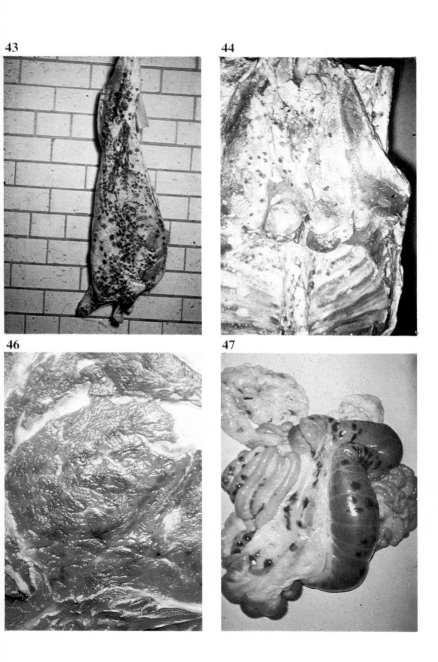

'BONE TAINT'

48. BOVINE HINDQUARTER. Note the discoloration (*arrow*) close to the bone.

BOWEL OEDEMA DISEASE

49. PIG. Note the oedematous swelling of the eyelids.

BRUISING

50. BOVINE CARCASE. This often occurs when an animal goes down in the transit vehicle, is unable to rise and is trampled on by the other animals, particularly when the vehicle is overloaded.

51. PIG CARCASE.

CALF DIPHTHERIA

52. CALF TONGUE. The causal organism is *Fusiformis necrophorus*. Note the large necrotic lesion. The lesions may also be found elsewhere in the mouth and pharynx. The condition only affects young calves.

CARCINOMA

53. SHEEP LIVER. Neoplastic conditions are uncommon in sheep.

48

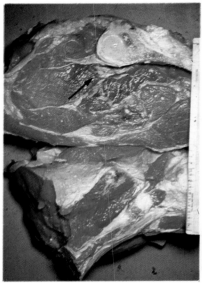

51

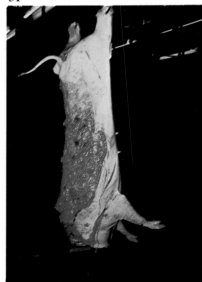

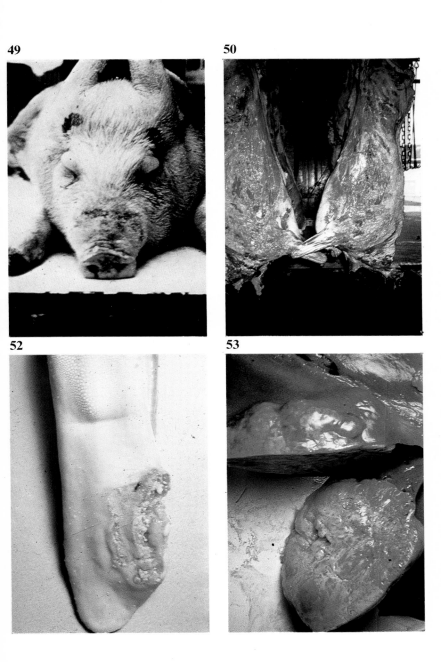

49

50

52

53

54

CARCINOMA, cont.

54. PIG LIVER. Note the similarity to the sheep liver in **53**.

CASEOUS LYMPHADENITIS

55. SHEEP LYMPH NODE. The causal organism is *Corynebacterium ovis* (*C. pseudotuberculosis,* bacillus Preisz-Nocard). This shows the typical onion-like appearance of the older lesion.

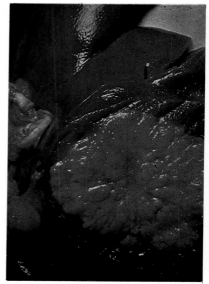

CHIARI'S DISEASE

56. BOVINE LIVER. The portal veins have been opened to show the typical pale thrombi (*arrows*). The cause is unknown.

CHONDROMA

57. SHEEP.

57

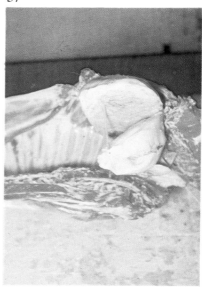

COENURUS CEREBRALIS

58. SHEEP BRAIN. This is the cystic stage of the dog tapeworm *Multiceps multiceps (Taenia multiceps)* which causes the disease 'gid' or 'sturdy'. The cyst has been opened to show the scolices (*arrow*).

59. SHEEP BRAIN. The scolices are much more numerous than in **58**. Cysts on the surface of the brain can soften the cranial bone.

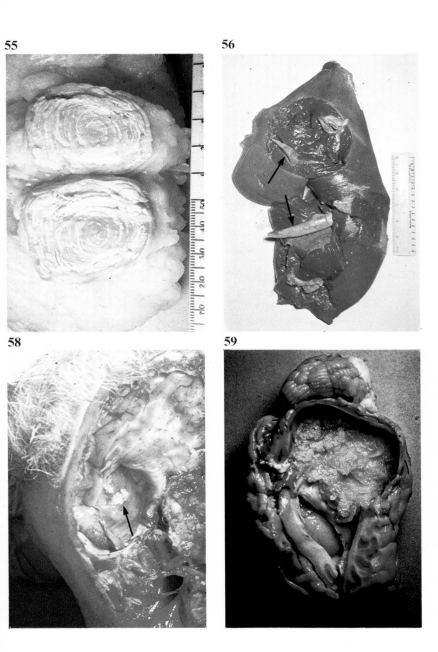

55

56

58

59

CORYNEBACTERIUM EQUI

60. PIG SUBMAXILLARY LYMPH NODE. The necrotic lesions have the appearance and consistency of white lead paint and shell out easily. The lesions greatly resemble those of avian tuberculosis (see **258**).

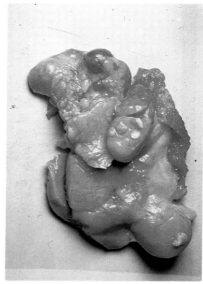

CYST (CONGENITAL)
61. PIG KIDNEY. These malformations occur during embryonic development.

62. SHEEP KIDNEY.

CYSTIC OVARY
63. BOVINE. This is a distention cyst which is a common cause of infertility.

64. PIG.

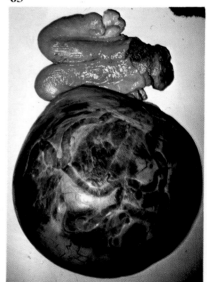

61

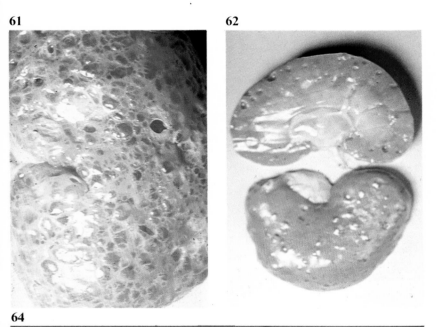

62

64

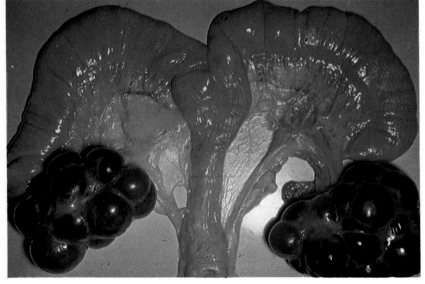

CYSTICERCUS BOVIS

65. BOVINE MASSETER MUSCLE. This is the cystic stage of the human tapeworm *Taenia saginata*. Viable cysts (*arrow*) are clear and the single scolex is visible in each.

66. BOVINE MASSETER MUSCLE. The degenerate cyst (*arrow*) is opaque.

67. BOVINE MASSETER MUSCLE. Two degenerate cysts are visible which show evidence of encapsulation and calcification. The disc measures 2cm across.

68. BOVINE LIVER. The cyst is viable and the scolex has evaginated probably due to the action of the bile from the liver. Cysts rarely develop in sites other than muscle.

69. BOVINE HEART. Numerous viable cysts are evident.

CYSTICERCUS CELLULOSAE

70. PIG MUSCLE. This is the cystic stage of the human tapeworm *Taenia solium*.

65

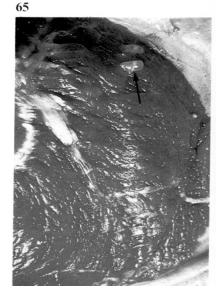

68

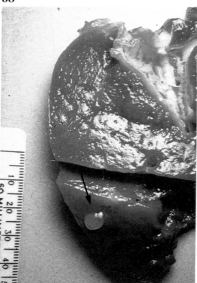

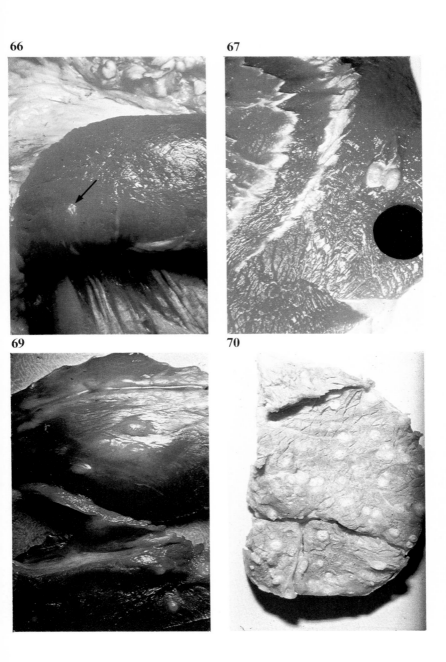

66   67

69   70

CYSTICERCUS OVIS

71. SHEEP HEART. This is the cystic stage of the dog tapeworm *Taenia ovis*. Predilection sites are the heart, diaphragm and masseter muscles.

72. SHEEP MUSCLE. This was from a generalised case in which the whole musculature was invaded.

CYSTICERCUS TENUICOLLIS

73. SHEEP LIVER. This is the cystic stage of the dog tapeworm *Taenia hydatigena*. The haemorrhagic tracks are freshly made by the larvae wandering through the liver.

74. SHEEP LIVER. The tracks have begun to caseate.

75. SHEEP LIVER. The tracks have become caseous. Note that the cysts are not in the liver substance but are on the peritoneal surface.

76. SHEEP LIVER. There are numerous cysts on the peritoneal surface of the liver. Some of the cysts have been evaginated, each showing a single scolex.

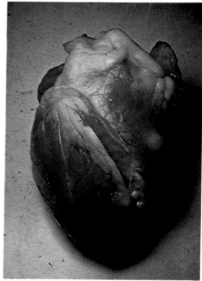

74

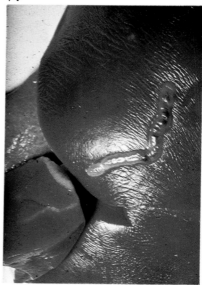

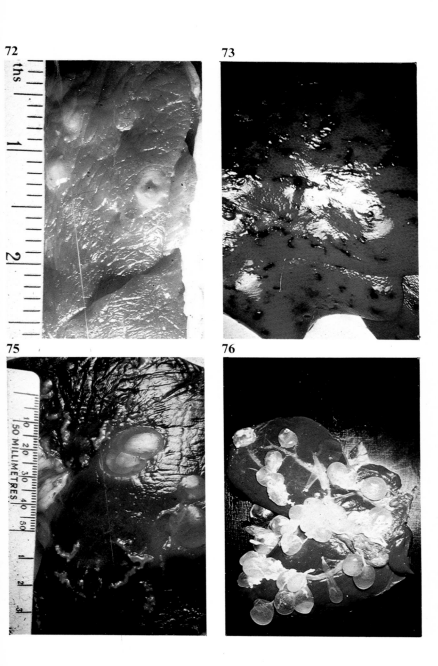

CYSTITIS

77. PIG BLADDER. Note the inflammatory nature of mucous membrane.

ECHINOCOCCUS (HYDATID) CYSTS

78. SHEEP LUNGS AND LIVER. This is the cystic stage of the dog tapeworm *Echinococcus granulosus*. The cysts are in the substance of the liver: compare with **75** and **76**. Note that there is no tissue reaction over the cysts due to the parasitic membrane being almost inert.

79. SHEEP LIVER. The cyst has been opened to show the very numerous scolices on the lining membrane.

80. SHEEP LEG.

81. BOVINE LIVER AND SPLEEN. The single cyst (*arrow*) is very large, a common feature in the spleen.

82. BOVINE LIVER. The degenerated cysts have caseous centres which are easily enucleated from the distinctly fibrous cyst walls.

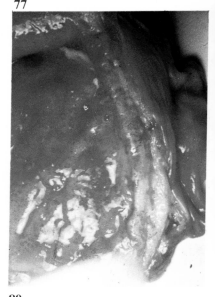

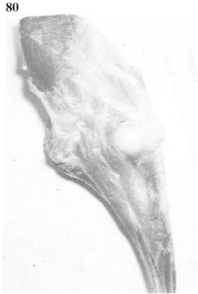

78

79

81

82

ECHINOCOCCUS (HYDATID) CYSTS, cont.

83. BOVINE KIDNEY. This can be distinguished from a retention cyst by the presence of the parasitic membrane.

84. BOVINE HEART. The cyst is arrowed.

85. PIG SPLEEN.

86. PIG LIVER. Endogenous daughter cysts. The large cyst has been opened to show the numerous daughter cysts. The formation of daughter cysts is often stimulated when the life of the original cyst is endangered.

87. HORSE LIVER. These cysts are believed to be the cystic stage of a sub-species *Echinococcus granulosus equinus* of which the dog is probably the definitive host. The cysts are very common in horses and show great variation in size.

ENTERITIS AND PERITONITIS
88. BOVINE INTESTINE.

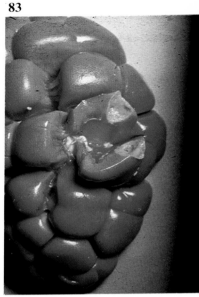

83

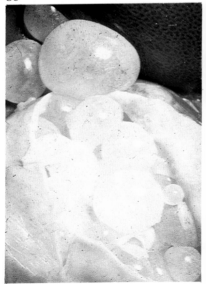

86

84

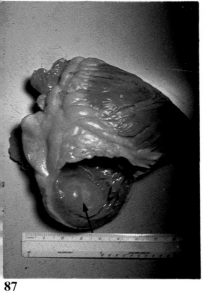

85

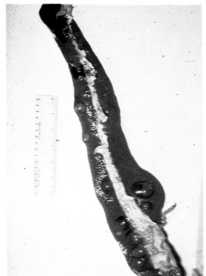

87

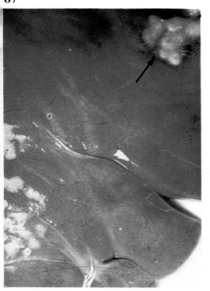

88

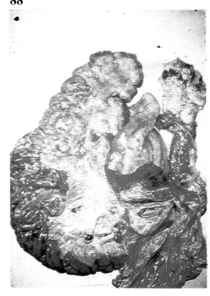

ENZOOTIC (VIRUS) PNEUMONIA

89. PIG LUNGS. The causal organism is *Mycoplasma suipneumoniae*. The lesions are generally confined to the edges of the apical and cardiac lobes. Note the inflammatory lymph nodes (*arrows*).

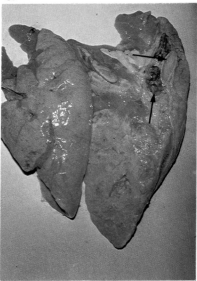

EOSINOPHILIC MYOSITIS

90. BOVINE MUSCLE. This shows as light green coloration of the muscle (*arrow*). The cause is unknown.

FASCIOLIASIS (FLUKY LIVER OR LIVER ROT)

91. SHEEP LIVER. The causal organism is *Fasciola hepatica* or liver fluke. The typical enlarged bile ducts which contain many worms are seen.

92. BOVINE LIVER. The bile ducts are markedly fibrous and contain black encrustations of calcium. The condition is that of a biliary cirrhosis. Two flukes from the opened bile ducts are visible on the surface.

92

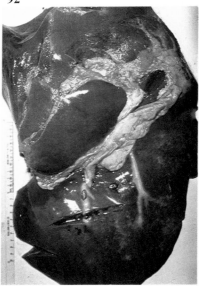

93. BOVINE LUNG. These cysts are found in the lungs, from about the size of a hazel nut up to 4 or 5cm, containing brownish detritus (*arrow*).

94. BOVINE LUNG. Note the one unopened cyst (A) and the opened cyst (B) showing the hard calcified cyst wall. The cysts are generally found towards the base of the lungs. There is little tissue reaction from the serous membrane.

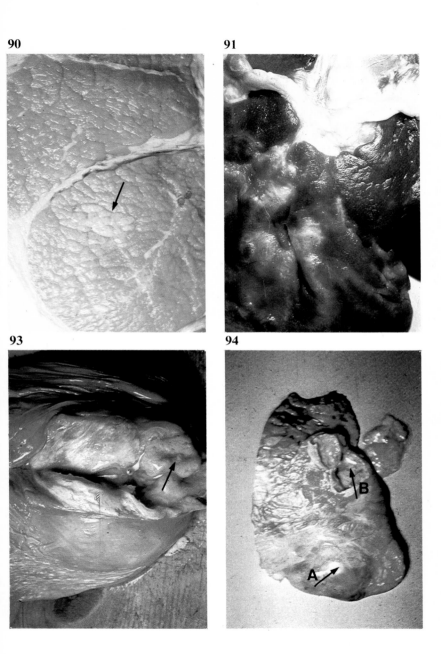

90

91

93

94

FASCIOLIASIS, cont.

95. BOVINE PERITONEUM. This is due to a very heavy infestation and migration of the immature flukes. The lesions have the typical greenish tinge.

96. PIG LIVER. Two flukes are arrowed. It is unusual to find pig livers infested, probably because of the method of husbandry. When damage does occur it resembles that of the bovine.

FAT NECROSIS

97. BOVINE FAT. The necrotic area (*arrow*) has a dead white appearance against the normal fat.

98. BOVINE ABDOMINAL FAT. The hard necrotic fat is constricting the intestine (*arrow*). This widespread necrosis of the abdominal fat occurs mainly in Channel Island cattle. The cause is unknown, and the results may be fatal. Disc = 2cm.

99. BOVINE ABDOMINAL FAT. As in **98** the hard abdominal fat has a constricting action, this time on the kidney (*arrow*) which has atrophied so that only a portion remains. This is also from a Channel Island breed.

100. PIG ABDOMINAL FAT. Leakage of pancreatic juice from the pancreas, which lies in a loop of the small intestine adjacent to the kidney, causes this fat necrosis. The small areas of necrosis show up well against the normal fat just below the disc (2cm across).

95

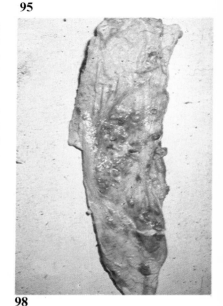

98

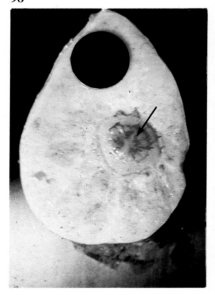

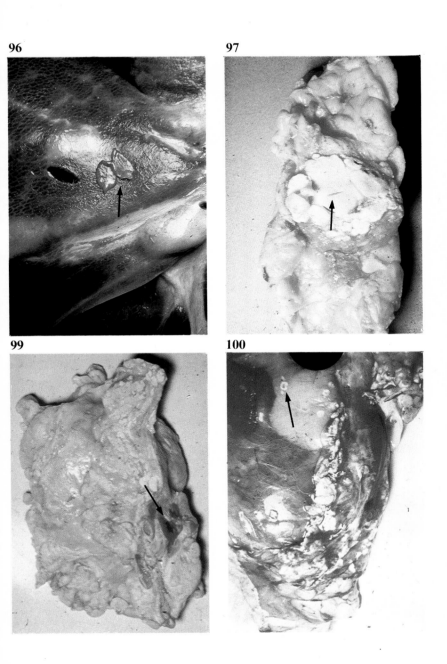

101

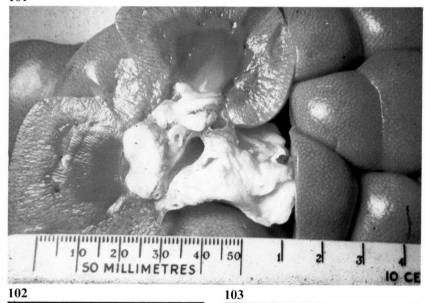

102

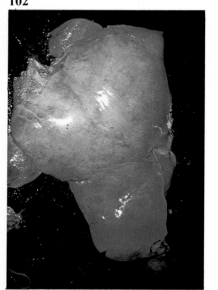

103

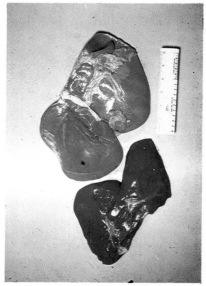

FATTY INFILTRATION

101. BOVINE KIDNEY.

102. BOVINE LIVER (SEE **12**). This is often brought about by a general-ised condition such as toxaemia.

103. SHEEP LIVER. The fatty liver is from a case of pregnancy toxaemia ('twin lamb disease'). A normal liver is shown below for comparison.

FEVERED CARCASE

104. BOVINE. This is a result of traumatic peritonitis and pleurisy. The muscles are dark and the whole carcase has a generally bright red appearance. There is an acute septic peritonitis with a large area of sepsis (*arrow*).

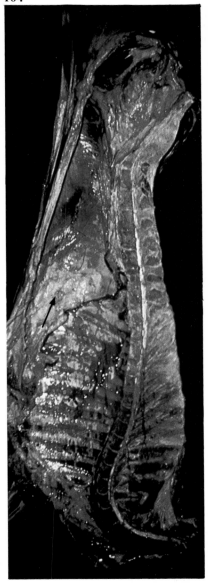

FIBROMA
105. SHEEP MAMMARY GLANDS.

106. SHEEP MAMMARY GLANDS (SAME SHEEP AS **105**). The tumour had grown through the skin and was heavily contaminated.

107. SHEEP TEAT.

FIBROPLASTIC NEPHRITIS (WHITESPOT)
108. CALF KIDNEY. The cause of this condition is unknown and is only found in calves up to about 10 months, indicating a spontaneous disappearance of the groups of endothelioid cells which make up the lesions.

FOOT AND MOUTH DISEASE
109. BOVINE TONGUE. The causal organism is a virus. There is an unruptured vesicle on the tongue.

110. BOVINE TONGUE. There is a ruptured vesicle on the dorsal prominence.

105

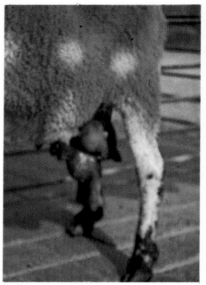

108

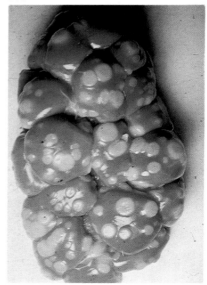

106

107

109

110

FOOT AND MOUTH DISEASE, cont.

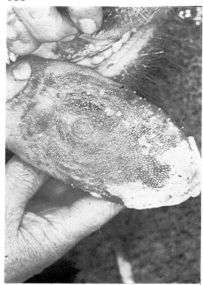

111. BOVINE TONGUE. The upper surface is denuded of epithelium except at the tip where necrotic epithelium still adheres.

112. BOVINE TEAT. A considerable area is denuded of epithelium. In places the epithelium is only partially detached. Healing has commenced.

113. SHEEP LIP. There is a ruptured vesicle on the commisure of the lower lip (*arrow*).

114. SHEEP FOOT. Interdigital cleft showing separation and under-running of the horn at the coronet.

115. SHEEP FOOT. There is separation of the horn at the coronet (*arrow*).

116. PIG TONGUE. There are two small rising vesicles on the tongue. The lesions are indistinguishable from those of swine vesicular disease (see **232**).

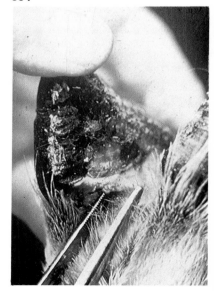

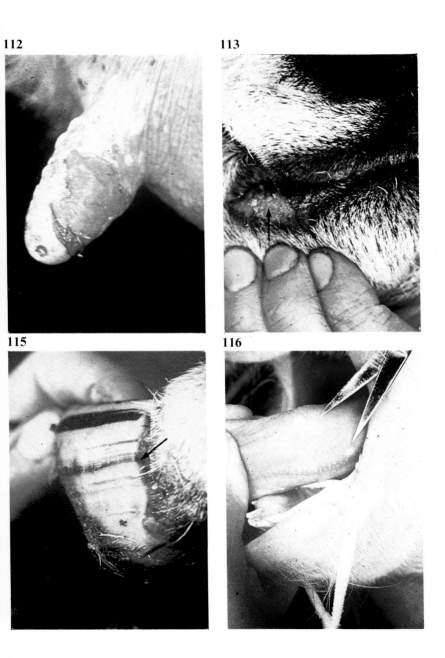

112

113

115

116

FOOT AND MOUTH DISEASE, cont.

117. PIG FOOT. There are ruptured vesicles on the main and supernumerary digits.

118. PIG FOOT. There are ruptured vesicles and separation of the horn extending all round the coronet.

FOREIGN BODY

119. PIG SPLEEN. A cocktail stick is seen penetrating the spleen (*arrow*). Sharp penetrating objects such as needles, pins, bristles of bass brooms etc are fairly common in the abdominal cavity of swill fed pigs.

120. PIG CAECUM. A bristle from a bass broom is penetrating the caecum.

FRACTURE

121. PIG VERTEBRAE. This injury is fairly common in pigs and probably occurs when the animal is very young when the sow may lie on its piglets. Note that the spinal cord is undamaged.

122. SHEEP VERTEBRAE. This is a similar condition to **121**. Note the good condition of the carcase indicating that the lesion had not disabled the animal.

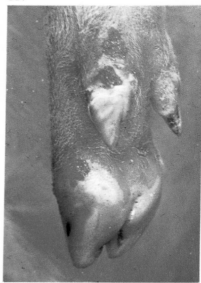

120

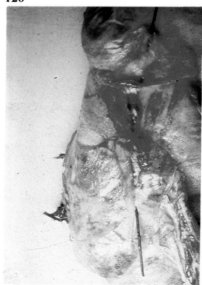

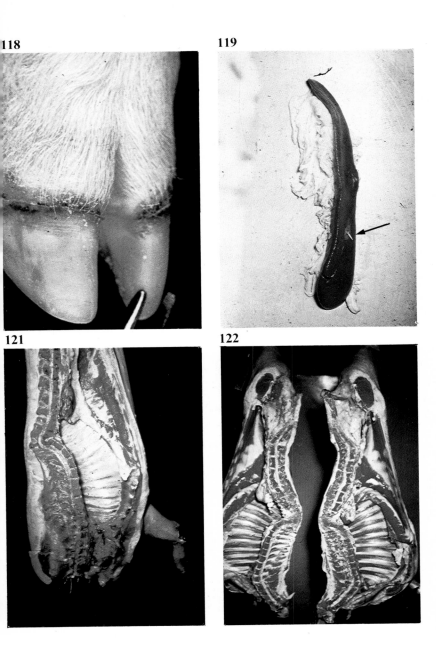

FRACTURE, cont.

123. SHEEP LEG. This probably occurred during transit to the abattoir. Fracture of tibia (A) and fracture of metatarsal (B).

FREEZER BURN

124. PIG KIDNEY . The areas of freezer burn are lighter in colour and are due to dehydration from excessive refrigeration.

GALL STONE

125. PIG. The wall of the gall bladder is thickened due to fibrosis caused by irritation. The disc measures 2cm across.

GANGRENE

126. SHEEP METATARSUS. The gangrene has followed a compound fracture.

'GOLDEN SLIPPERS'

127. BOVINE FOETAL FEET. Note the yellow colour and also that the soles are convex.

123

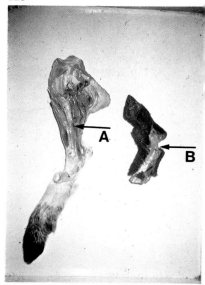

126

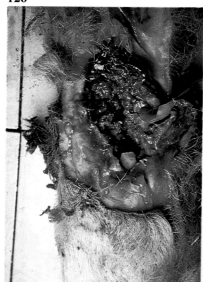

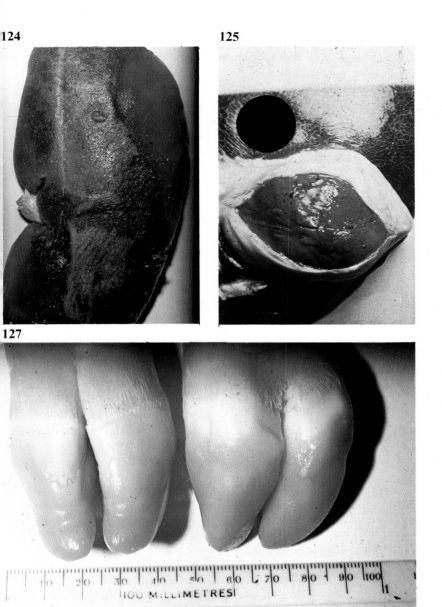

124

125

127

HAIR BALL

128. BOVINE. This is a cross section of a hair ball from the rumen showing closely packed hairs. The hard outer cover is composed of a deposit of salts.

129. PIG STOMACH.

HEPATITIS (CHRONIC)

130. BOVINE LIVER.

131. BOVINE LIVER. This is a cross section of **130**.

HEPATITIS (MULTILOBULAR CIRRHOSIS, 'HOBNAIL LIVER')

132. BOVINE LIVER. New islands of liver tissue develop as a compensatory hypertrophy.

133. BOVINE LIVER. This is similar to the liver in **132** but more advanced.

128

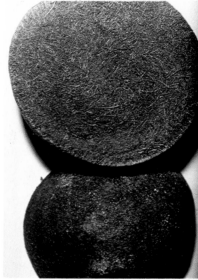

131

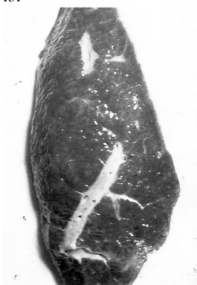

129

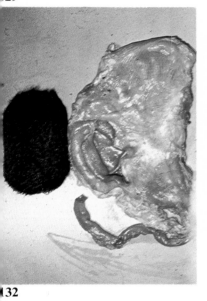

130

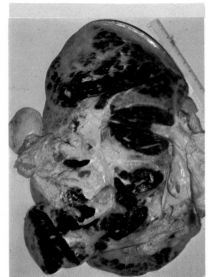

132

133

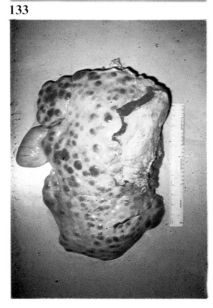

HYALINE DEGENERATION
134. BOVINE MUSCLE. Areas of degeneration are seen at A and B.

HYDROCEPHALUS
135. CALF.

HYDRONEPHROSIS
136. BOVINE KIDNEY. Only a few lobules are involved. This is caused by obstruction to the outflow of urine.

137. BOVINE KIDNEY. All the lobules are involved and practically no kidney substance remains. This is an example of atrophy. In some cases such kidneys can weigh more than 40kg. Very often there is compensatory hypertrophy of the other kidney.

138. PIG KIDNEY.

134

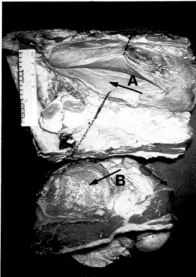

136

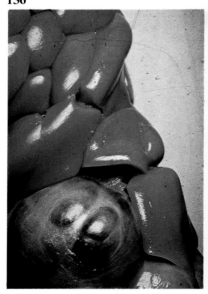

135

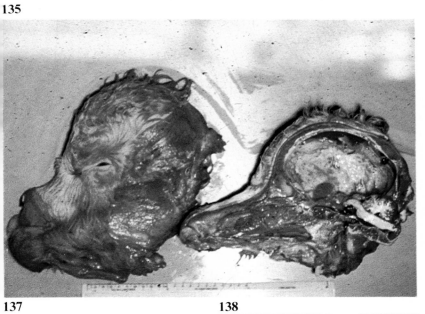

137

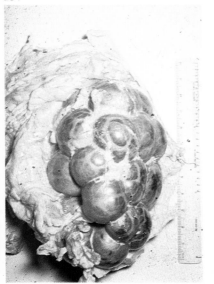

138

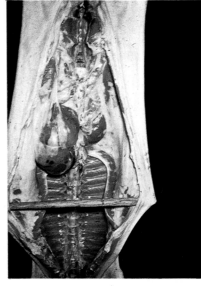

HYDRONEPHROSIS, cont.
139. PIG KIDNEY.

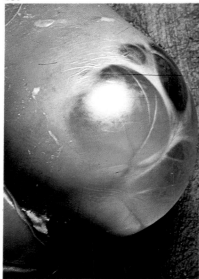

HYOSTRONGYLUS RUBIDUS NODULES
140. PIG STOMACH. The larvae pene-
trate into the pits of the gastric
glands until they become adults.
They may remain there for several
months causing the formation of
the nodules.

INFARCTS
141. BOVINE KIDNEY. These are
due to occlusion of capillaries by
thrombi leading to necrosis and
eventually fibrosis.

INSUFFIENCY OF BLEEDING
142. SHEEP LUNGS. The lungs are
dark red and contain a large
amount of blood. There is an
accompanying fatty infiltration of
the liver caused by toxaemia which
also accounted for the bad bleeding.

143. SHEEP. Note that the capillaries
on the back of the sheep are plainly
seen and are full of blood.

JAUNDICE
144. CALF. Note the general yellow
colour of the fat, ribs and particularly the abdominal aorta (*arrow*).

142

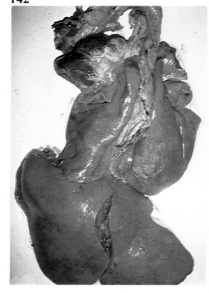

140

141

143

144

JAUNDICE, cont.
145. PIG. Note the yellow colour of the skin.

146. PIG. Note the yellow colour of the fat, especially the peritoneal ('leaf') fat and the yellow colour of the ribs.

JÖHNES DISEASE
147. BOVINE INTESTINES ('THICK ROPES'). The causal organism is *Mycobacterium jöhnei*. Note the haemorrhagic corrugations in the opened intestines. Ulceration is mechanical as the corrugations impinge on one another.

LUNG WORMS (PARASITIC PNEUMONIA, HOOSE OR HUSK)
148. BOVINE LUNG. The causal organism is *Dictyocaulus viviparus*. Note the worms lying in an opened bronchiole (*arrow*).

149. SHEEP LUNGS. The cause here is *Dictyocaulus filaria*. Note the localised areas of pneumonia and the emphysema caused by the blockage of the bronchioles.

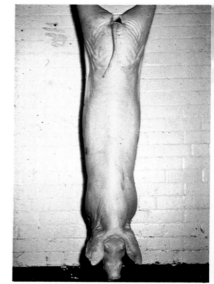

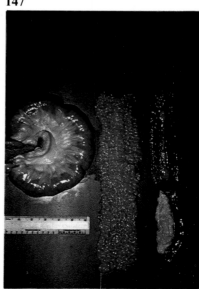

146

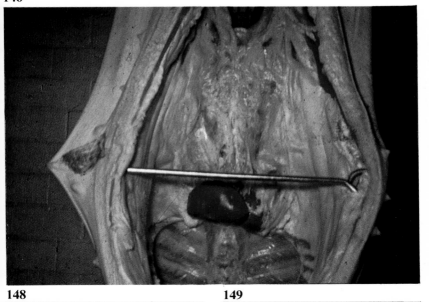

148

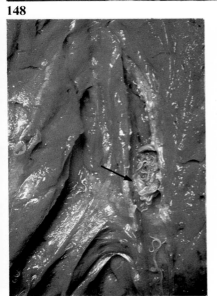

149

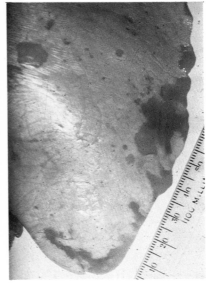

LUNG WORMS, cont.

150. SHEEP LUNGS. The cause is *Dictyocaulus filaria*. Note the local patches of emphysema at a later stage than **149**.

151. SHEEP LUNGS. The cause is *Muellerius capillaris*, by far the commonest lung worm in sheep. It produces the greyish nodule. The mediastinal lymph nodes are also affected (*arrow*). Lesions in younger sheep are pearly white and are caused by *Protostrongylus rufescens*.

152. PIG LUNG. The cause is *Metastrongylus apri*. Note the well defined pearl coloured emphysematous plaque (*arrow*) due to blockage of a bronchiole.

153. PIG LUNG. Caused by *Metastrongylus apri*. Note the well defined emphysematous plaque which has been cut through.

LYMPHOSARCOMA

154. SHEEP CARCASE AND OFFAL. The causal organism is a virus.

150

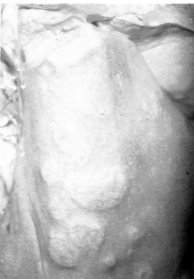

152

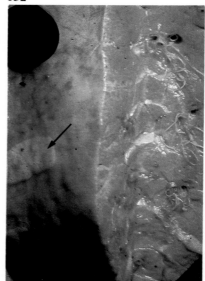

151

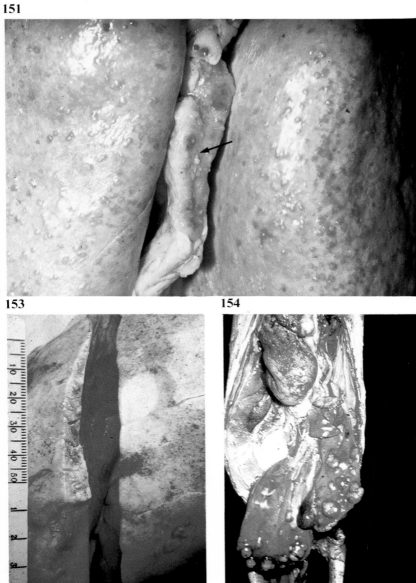

153

154

LYMPHOSARCOMA, cont.

155. SHEEP KIDNEY, LIVER AND LUNG.

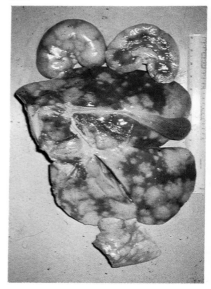

156. BOVINE CARCASE. Note the large and numerous tumours (A) in the lungs which are hanging from an S-hook in the flank. Large and inflammatory lesions are obvious at the abdominal entrance of the pelvis (B).

157. PIG CARCASE. Note the large and inflammatory internal iliac lymph node (A) and the lumbar lymph nodes (B).

MACERATED FOETUS
158. BOVINE. See also **170**.

MAGGOT INFECTION
159. SHEEP SUBCUTANEOUS TISSUE. The larva of the sheep maggot fly (*Lucilia sericata*) is seen at A. Note the burrow hole at B.

MELANOMA
160. CALF SKIN.

158

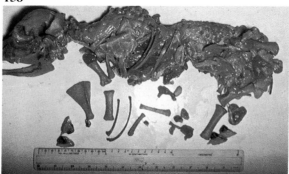

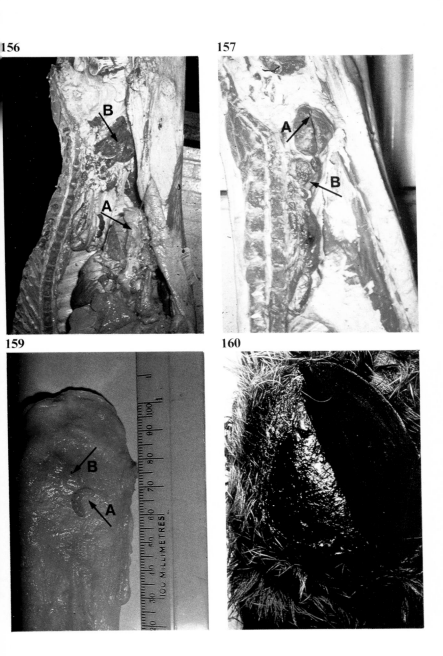

MELANOMA, cont.
161. PIG SKIN.

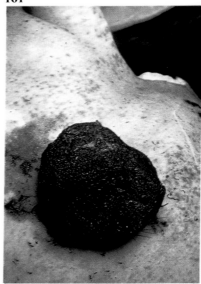

MELANOSIS
162. PIG SKIN. A piece of the rind has been stripped off to show the normal subcutaneous fat. The white patches are normal coloured skin.

163. PIG MAMMARY TISSUE ('SEEDY CUT' OR 'SEEDY BELLY'). This condition occurs only in pigs with some black pigmented hairs and not in breeds such as Large Whites or Landraces.

164. SHEEP CARCASE AND OFFAL. The melanosis is present in the lungs, ribs and spinal cord (*arrow*).

MELANOSIS, cont.
165. CALF HEAD. Note that it is the periosteum which is affected.

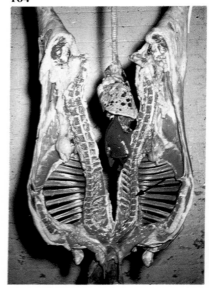

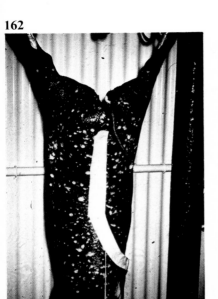

162

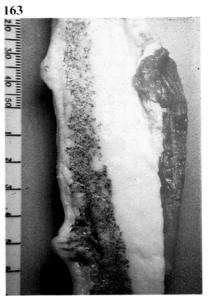

163

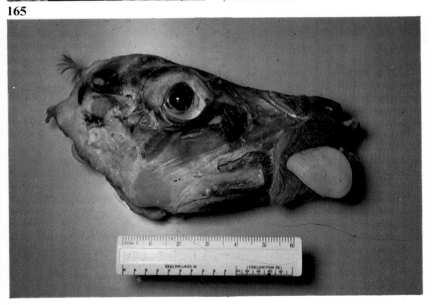

165

166. BOVINE LUNG. The texture of the lung is not altered, only the colour.

167. BOVINE SPINAL CORD. A normal cord is shown on the right for comparison. Note that it is the covering not the substance of the cord that is affected. The condition is often referred to as 'black pith'.

MENINGITIS (SEPTIC SPINAL)
168. PIG. Note the pus (*arrow*) in the spinal canal.

MESENTERIC (INTESTINAL) EMPHYSEMA
169. PIG. Numerous vesicles have formed, some of which are haemorrhagic. They burst on slight pressure. The cause is unknown.

MUMMIFIED FOETUS
170. BOVINE. See also **158**. The foetus may have died in the uterus some months before reaching this stage. The foetal fluid has been absorbed.

NECROBACILLOSIS (BACILLARY NECROSIS)
171. BOVINE LIVER. The causal organism is *Fusiformis necrophorus*. A feature of this condition is that all the lesions are about the same size – 3cm in diameter. The lesions consist of necrotic centres with haemorrhagic outer rings.

166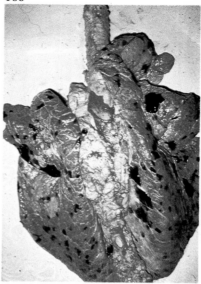

169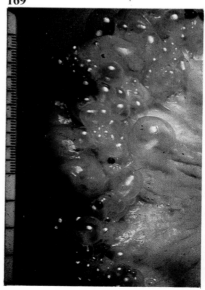

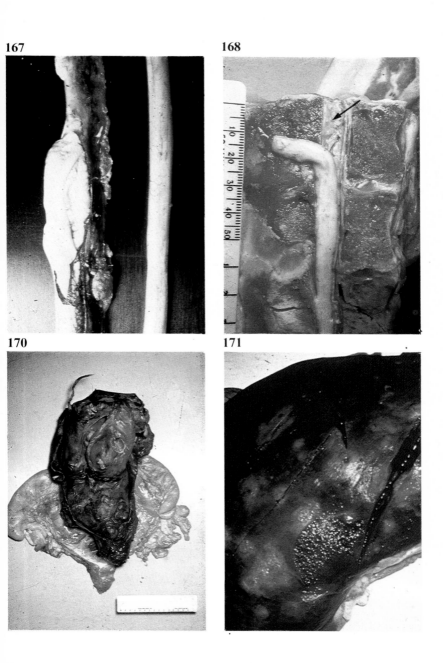

167

168

170

171

NECROBACILLOSIS, cont.

172. BOVINE LIVER. This is of a more chronic type than **171**.

NECROSIS

173. PIG TAIL. This is a result of the constriction due to the rubber band (*arrow*).

174. PIG TAIL. This is the result of 'tail biting'. The sequelae are very often abscesses in the pelvic region and vertebrae etc (see **5**).

NEPHRITIS (ACUTE)

175. PIG KIDNEY. The kidney is bright red in appearance and mottled. (Disc = 2cm across.)

NEPHRITIS (CHRONIC)

176. BOVINE KIDNEY. A normal kidney is shown for comparison. Note the enlargement, pale colour and pitted surface. The condition is often bilateral.

177. SHEEP KIDNEY. Note the pitted surface. The capsule is difficult to strip off.

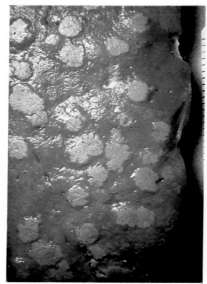

175

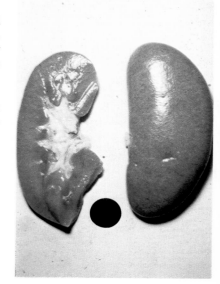

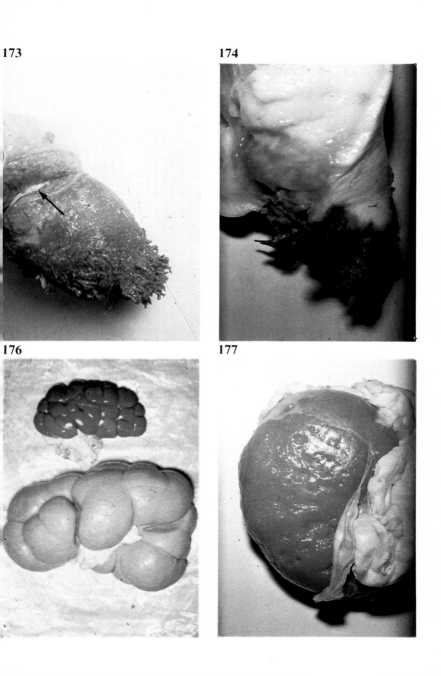

173

174

176

177

NEPHRITIS (CHRONIC), cont.

178. PIG KIDNEY. A normal kidney is shown for comparison. Note the pale colour and the roughened, pitted surface.

179. PIG KIDNEY. The surface is scarred and rough.

NEW FOREST DISEASE (INFECTIOUS KERATITIS)

180. BOVINE EYE. The causal organism is *Moraxella bovis*.

NODULAR NECROSIS (ROEKL'S GRANULOMA)

181. BOVINE TAIL AND NECK MUSCLE. The cause is unknown.

OEDEMA

182. SHEEP CARCASE. The carcase has a wet appearance and the kidney fat has not set. The condition is to be distinguished from a poor carcase which would set and not be dropsical.

183. SHEEP HEART. The fat on the heart has not set and has a gelatinous appearance and consistency.

178

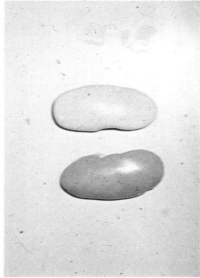

181

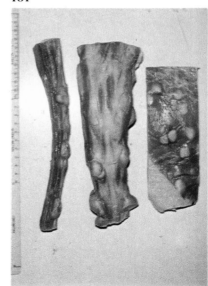

179

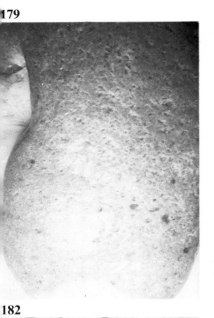

180

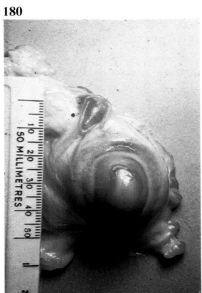

182

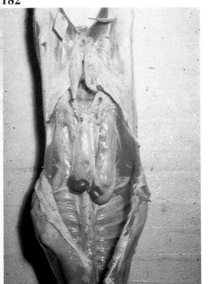

183

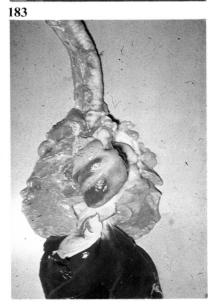

ORF (CONTAGIOUS PUS-TULAR DERMATITIS)

184. SHEEP. The causal organism is a virus. Note the lesions around the mouth area. Compare with foot and mouth vesicles in **113**.

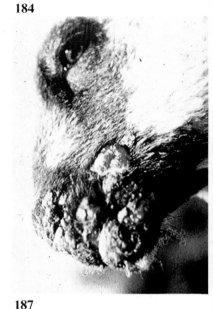

OSTEOHAEMATOCHROMA-TOSIS

185. CALF. The bones and kidneys are dark brown. Muscle has been stripped off to show the left tibia (*arrow*). The cause in unknown.

186. CALF. Various bones and kidney from **185**. Note that the cartilage still has the normal colour.

OSTEOMALACIA

187. BOVINE STERNUM. The bone marrow is dark red and has a jelly-like consistency.

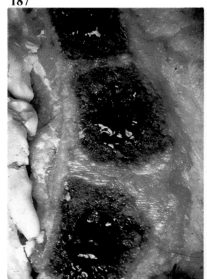

PANCREATIC CALCULI

188. BOVINE PANCREAS. The cause is unknown.

PAPILLOMA

189. BOVINE SKIN.

185

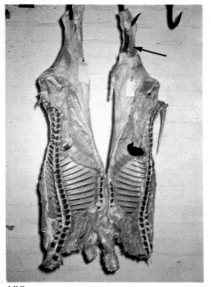

186

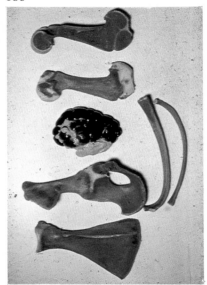

188

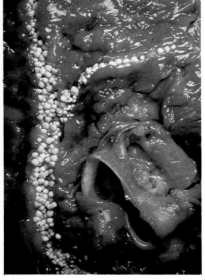

189

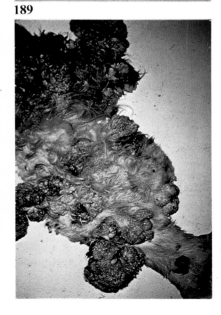

PENTASTOME LARVAE

190. BOVINE MESENTERIC LYMPH NODES. These are the lesions caused by the larvae of *Linguatula serrata*. The lesions are similar to tuberculosis but have a greenish tinge, and can occur in other organs in cattle and also sheep.

PERIARTERITIS NODOSA (POLYARTERITIS)

191. BOVINE HEART. This is a rare condition which results in nodular thickenings along the arteries.

PERICARDITIS

192. PIG HEART. Note the growth on the visceral pericardium and the very thickened pericardial sac.

PERICARDITIS AND OEDEMA

193. SHEEP HEART.

PERITONITIS (see also ENTERITIS)

194. PIG.

PIMPLY GUT

195. BOVINE INTESTINE. The nodules are caused by the penetration into the wall of the intestine by the larvae of *Oesophagostomum radiatum*.

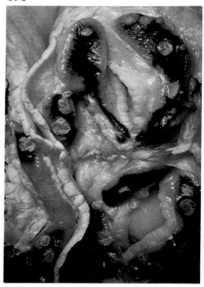

190

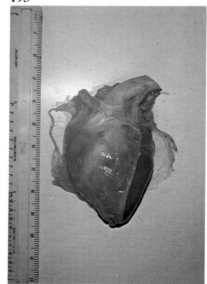

193

191

192

194

195

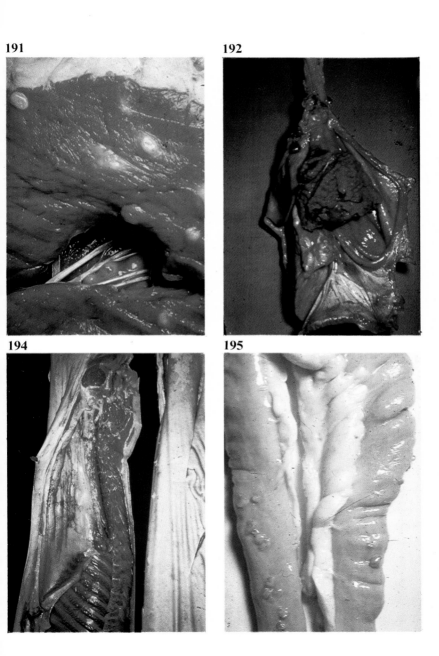

PIMPLY GUT, cont.

196. SHEEP INTESTINE. Nodules caused by the larvae of *Oesophagostomum columbianum*.

PLEURISY

197. PIG.

PNEUMONIA (see also ENZOOTIC PNEUMONIA)

198. LAMB LUNGS.

PORPHYRIA (CONGENITAL)

199. CALF KIDNEYS. Note the almost black colour of the kidneys and the brown colour of the kidney fat. The cause is unknown.

PRESTERNAL CALCIFICATION ('PUTTY BRISKET')

200. BOVINE. This is a pressure necrosis (*arrow*) of the fat which eventually calcifies. It only affects the fat and not the sternum.

196

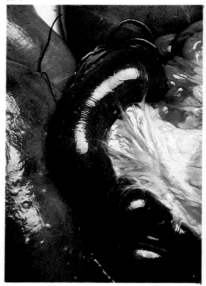

199

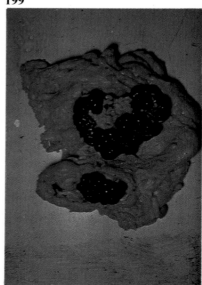

197

198

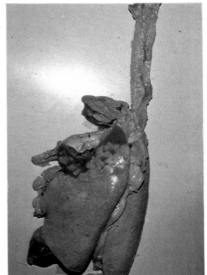

200

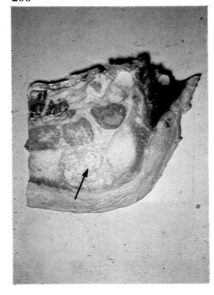

PRESTERNAL CALCIFICATION, cont.
201. BOVINE.

PYELONEPHRITIS
202. BOVINE KIDNEY. The causal organism is *Corynebacterium renale*. The kidney has a slate blue colour and the ureter (A) is very much enlarged as is also the renal lymph node (B).

203. BOVINE KIDNEY. The ureter is very much enlarged.

PYOMETRA
204. HORSE UTERUS.

RENAL CALCULI
205. SHEEP KIDNEY.

RINGWORM
206. CALF HEAD. The causal organism is *Trichophyton verrucosum*.

201

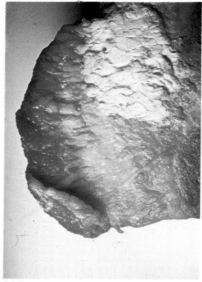

204

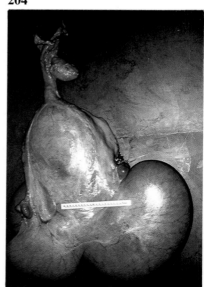

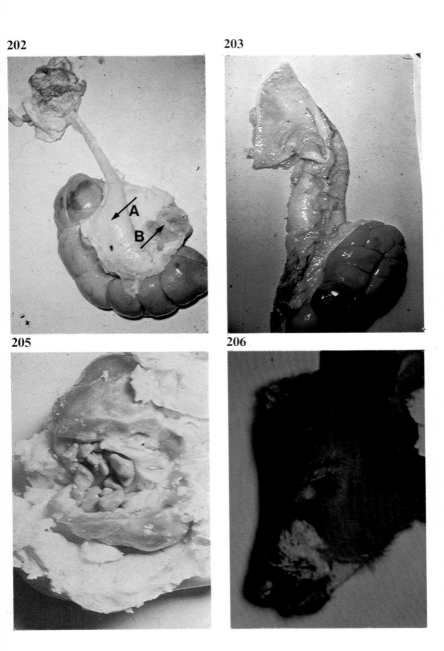

202

203

205

206

SARCOCYSTS (MIESCHER'S TUBES)

207. BOVINE MUSCLE. The organism is *Sarcocystis fusiformis*. The lesions are seen as small white circumscribed areas. They are usually smaller than *C. bovis* (see **67**).

208. PIG MUSCLE. The organism is *Sarcocystis miescheriana*.

209. SHEEP OESOPHAGUS. The organism is *Sarcocystis tenella*. The cysts are always large in this situation.

210. SHEEP HEART. The organism is *Sarcocystis tenella*.

211. SHEEP MUSCLE. The organism is *Sarcocystis tenella*.

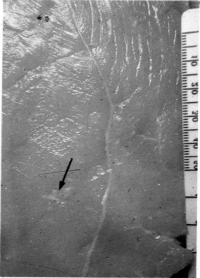

'SAWDUST LIVER' (FOCAL NECROSIS OF LIVER)

212. BOVINE LIVER. The condition is so-called because the lesions resemble sawdust scattered throughout the liver. The cause is bacterial in origin.

210

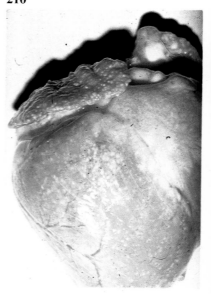

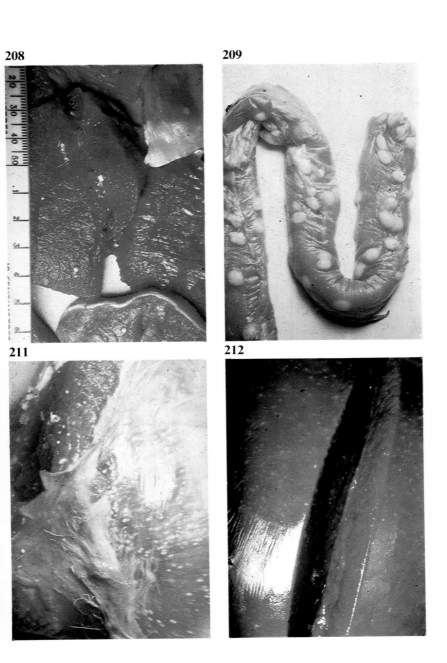

208

209

211

212

SHOTTY ERUPTION (SOOTY MANGE)

213. PIG SKIN. This often affects the skin of the buttocks when the patches are often symmetrical. The skin around the teats is also another common site. The cause is unknown.

STEATOSIS (INTERSTITIAL MYOSITIS, MUSCULAR FIBROSIS, LIPOMATOSIS OF MUSCLE)

214. PIG MUSCLE.

215. BOVINE MUSCLE. The muscle (A and B) has been completely replaced by the new tissue without any alteration in the gross shape of the muscle. The cause is unknown.

216. SHEEP MUSCLE. The muscles (A and B) have been replaced by the new fatty fibrous tissue.

'STICK MARKS'

217. PIG SKIN. The animal has been beaten with a stick, causing wheals. Compare with 'teeth marks' (**235**).

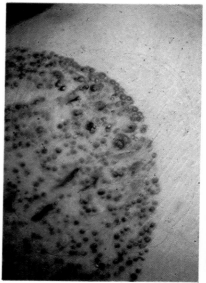

213

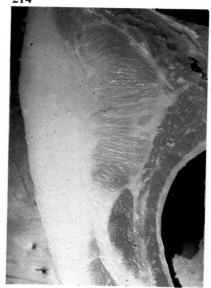

214

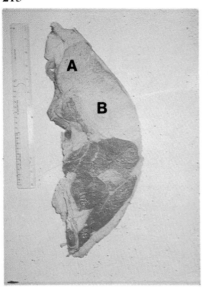

215

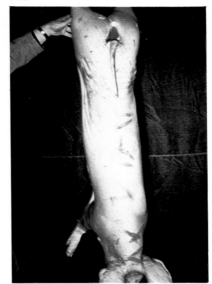

217

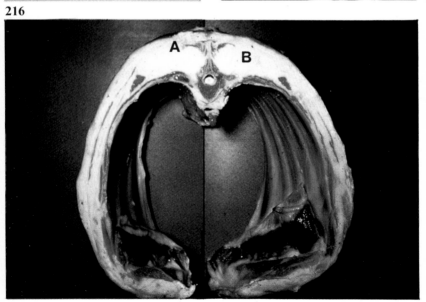

216

SWINE ERYSIPELAS URTICARIA ('DIAMONDS')

218. PIG SKIN. The causal organism is *Erysipelothrix rhusiopathiae*. During life the lesions are purplish in colour. However, after scalding they become red or brown.

SWINE ERYSIPELAS (VERRUCOSE ENDOCARDITIS)

219. PIG HEART. The vegetations have formed on the valves of the heart. Similar lesions can be caused by streptococci.

220. PIG LUNGS. This is the result of a verrucose endocarditis and shows the typical perilobular congestion.

221. PIG LUNG. A close-up shows the perilobular congestion.

222. PIG KIDNEY. Note the large infarcts (verrucae) and haemorrhages caused by emboli from the vegetations on the heart valves in verrucose endocarditis.

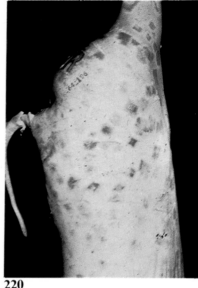

218

220

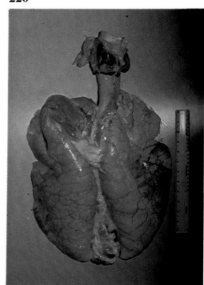

219

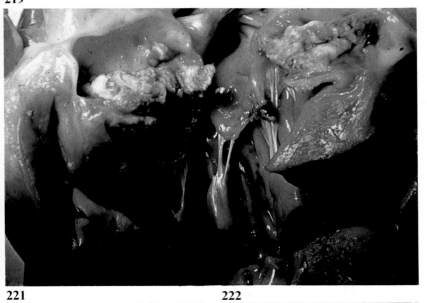

221

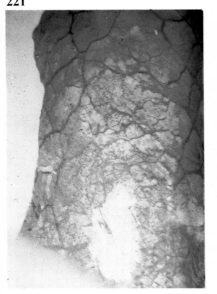

222

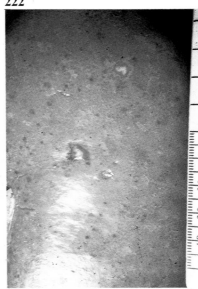

SWINE ERYSIPELAS, cont.

223. PIG STIFLE JOINT. This shows the typical chronic arthritis. Note the very inflammatory synovial membranes which produce the dark red or brown synovial fluid.

SWINE FEVER

224. PIG SKIN. The causal organism is a virus. Note the typical skin rash, especially on the ears.

225. PIG KIDNEY. The dark red petechial haemorrhages are typical of swine fever.

226. PIG KIDNEY AND LYMPH NODES. Note the typical dark haemorrhages in the kidneys and the inflammatory lymph nodes, dark at the periphery and pale in the centre.

227. PIG HEART. Note the typical petechial haemorrhages in the epicardium.

228. PIG INTESTINE. The typical 'button ulcers' have coalesced to form long lesions. A common secondary invader in this situation is *Salmonella choleraesuis*.

223

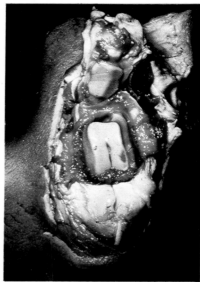

226

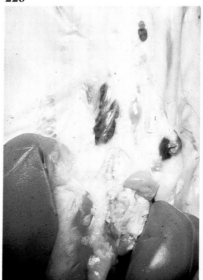

224

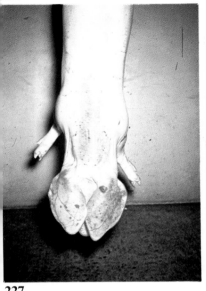

225

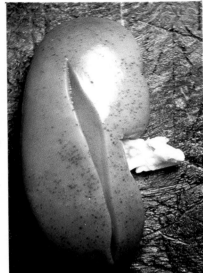

227

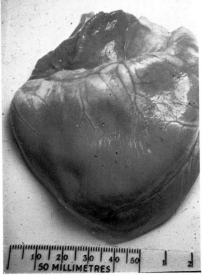

228

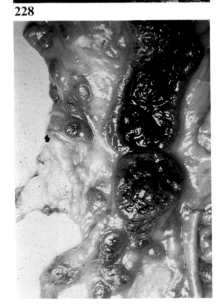

SWINE FEVER, cont.

229. PIG CAECUM. Note the typical 'button ulcers'. Compare with the normal caecum on the right which shows the ileo-caecal valve and Peyer's patches.

SWINE POX

230. PIG SKIN. The causal organism is a virus.

231. PIG SKIN. The disc measures 2cm across.

SWINE VESICULAR DISEASE

232. PIG FOOT. The causal organism is a virus. Note the ruptured vesicle on the bulb of the heel (*arrow*) and the scabbing of the leg lesions.

233. PIG SNOUT. Note the unruptured vesicle on the snout (*arrow*). The lesions in swine vesicular disease are indistinguishable from those of foot and mouth disease (see **116**).

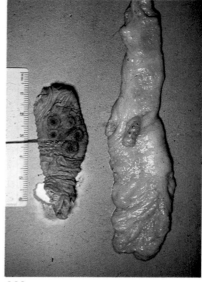

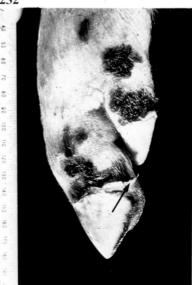

230

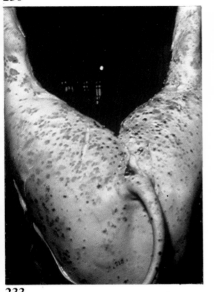

231

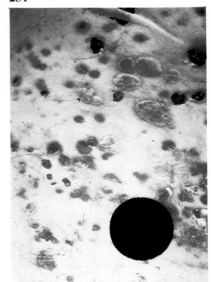

233

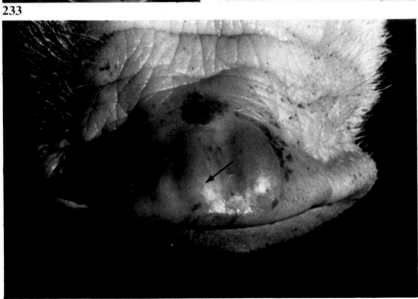

SWINE VESICULAR DISEASE, cont.

234. PIG FOOT. The soles of the digits have been shed showing the underlying tissue.

'TEETH MARKS'

235. PIG SKIN. These marks are due to fighting. Compare with 'stick marks' (**217**).

TELANGIECTASIS (CAVERNOUS HAEMANGIOMA, ANGIOMA)

236. BOVINE LIVER. This is common in the livers of old cows.

237. PIG LIVER. This condition is rare in pigs.

TORSION

238. PIG SPERMATIC CORD. Note the torsion (*arrow*) of the spermatic cord of the undescended testicle (cryptorchid pig) which has caused severe congestive enlargement of the testicle.

TRANSIT ERYTHEMA

239. PIG SKIN. This is a very severe case and the lesions on the left hind leg (A) and left fore leg (B) are commoner. The skin inflammation is due to irritation by urine or disinfectants.

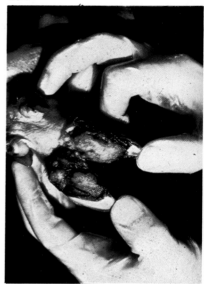

234

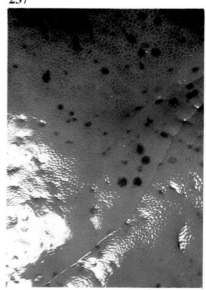

237

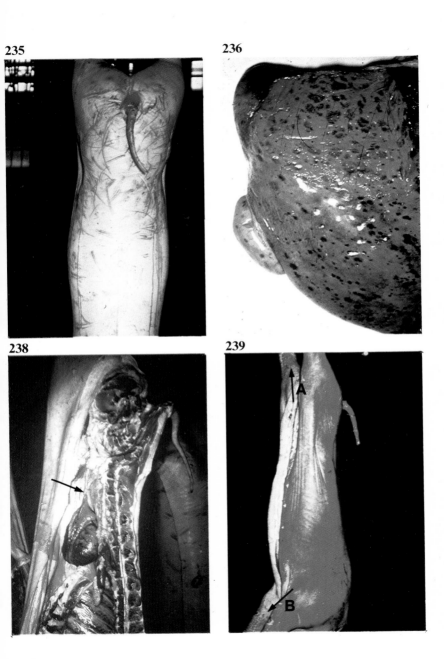

235

236

238

239

TRAUMATIC PERICARDITIS

240. BOVINE. Note the septic pericarditis caused by the penetration of a nail or wire from the reticulum carrying with it pyogenic organisms.

241. BOVINE. Note the adhesions to the thoracic wall (*arrow*).

242. BOVINE. Note the septic pleurisy and the penetration fistula through the diaphragm (*arrow*).

243. BOVINE. Severe septic peritonitis and pleurisy due to a foreign body. Note the penetration fistula through the diaphragm (*arrow*). The carcase is fevered.

TRAUMATIC RETICULITIS

244. BOVINE RETICULUM. This shows penetration by a wire.

240

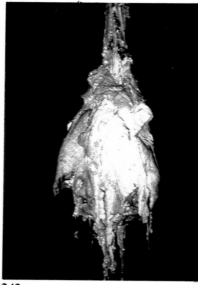

242

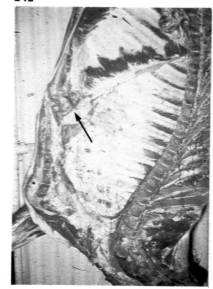

241

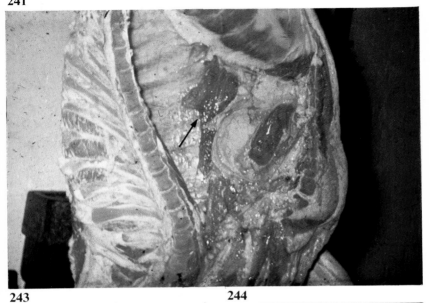

243

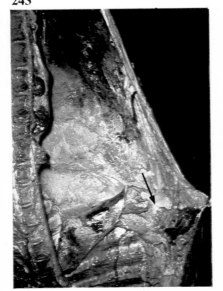

244

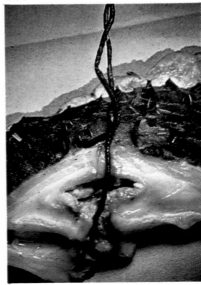

TRICHINOSIS

245. MUSCLE. The cause is *Trichinella spiralis*. This is a section of muscle showing the parasitic cyst. The actual size of the cyst is approximately 0.25 × 0.5mm.

TUBERCULOSIS

246. CALF CARCASE AND OFFAL (CONGENITAL TUBERCULOSIS). The causal organism is *Mycobacterium bovis* (*M. tuberculosis*, bovine strain). The liver is suspended from an S-hook.

247. BOVINE LUNG. The substance of the lung is affected.

248. BOVINE TRACHEA. Note the lesions on the mucous membrane and in the wall as indicated by the arrows.

249. BOVINE PERICARDIUM. The pericardial sac is held open by skewers.

250. BOVINE PERITONEUM. Acute tuberculosis is shown by the inflammatory velvety growth on the peritoneum. Compare with actinobacillosis of the peritoneum (**24**).

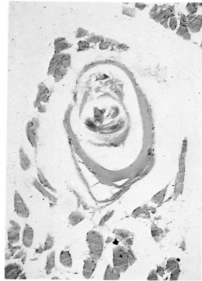

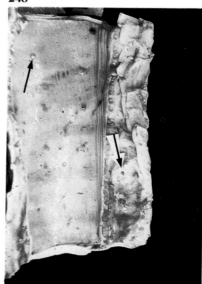

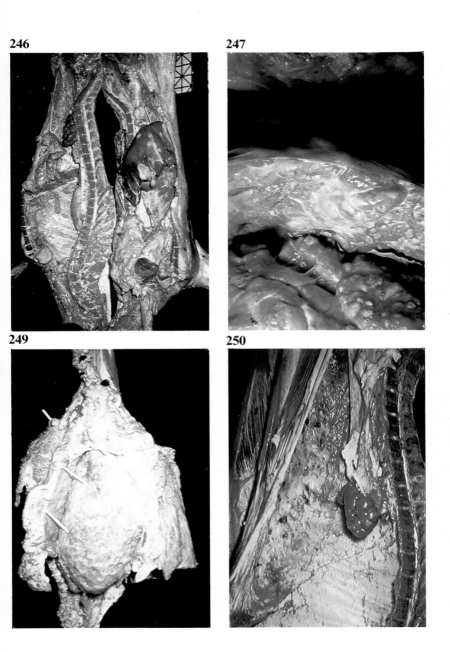

TUBERCULOSIS, cont.

251. BOVINE LIVER. This is an example of chronic tuberculosis.

252. BOVINE LIVER. Note the absence of white fibrous tissue and compare with actinobacillosis of the liver (**22**).

253. BOVINE LIVER (MILIARY TUBERCULOSIS). Note the similarity in the size of the tuberculosis nodules and the even distribution.

254. BOVINE KIDNEY.

255. BOVINE SPLEEN.

256. BOVINE SPINAL CORD.

251

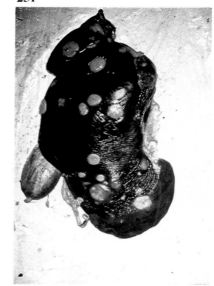

254

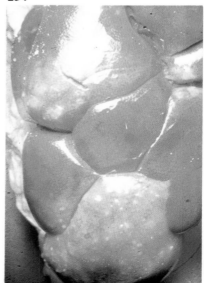

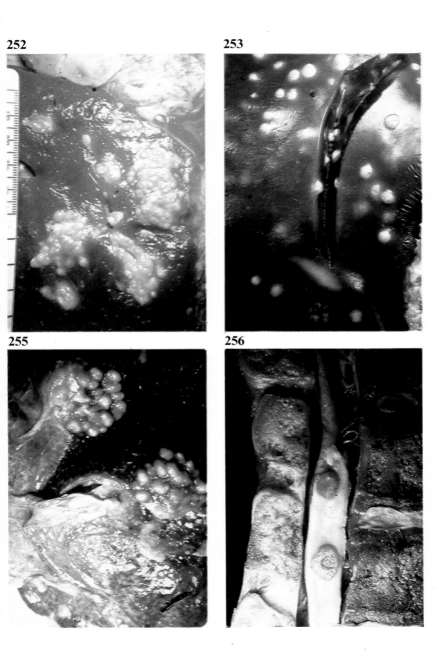

252

253

255

256

TUBERCULOSIS, cont.
257. BOVINE STERNUM.

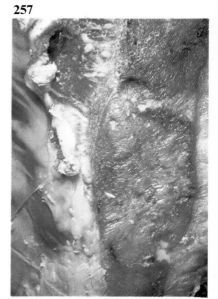

257

TUBERCULOSIS (AVIAN)
258. PIG SUBMAXILLARY LYMPH NODE. The causal organism is *Mycobacterium avium* (*M. tuberculosis,* avian strain). The lesions can be like those caused by *Corynebacterium equi* (see **60**).

TUBERCULOSIS (BOVINE)
259. PIG LYMPH NODES. The lesions are much more active and inflammatory than those caused by the avian strain (see **258**).

260. PIG MESENTERIC LYMPH NODES. The lesions have almost entirely calcified.

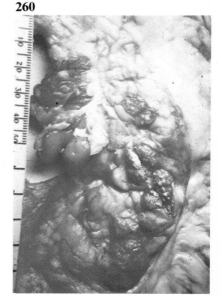

260

261. PIG LUNGS, LIVER AND SPLEEN. This is miliary tuberculosis. The lesions in the lungs are difficult to see but can be felt easily by palpation.

258

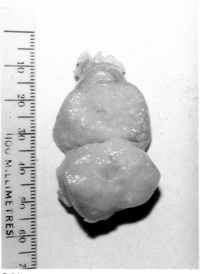

259

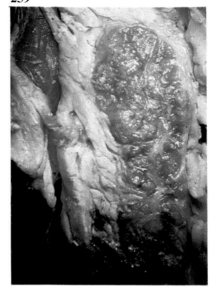

261

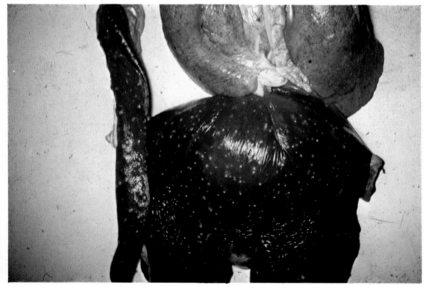

TUBERCULOSIS (BOVINE), cont.

262. PIG LIVER.

263. PIG HIP JOINT.

264. PIG HIP JOINT. This is a close-up of the femur in **263** showing tuberculosis lesions in the substance of the bone (*arrow*).

265. PIG HIP JOINT. These are the bones from **263** showing erosion of the head of the femur and pelvic bones.

266. HORSE LUNG. This is a miliary tuberculosis.

267. HORSE LIVER. Miliary tuberculosis.

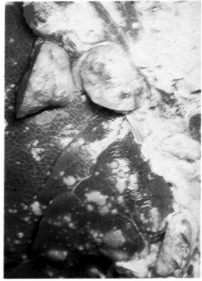

262

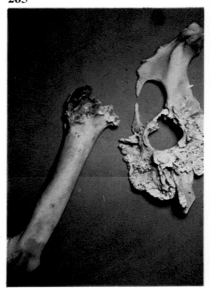

265

263

264

266

267

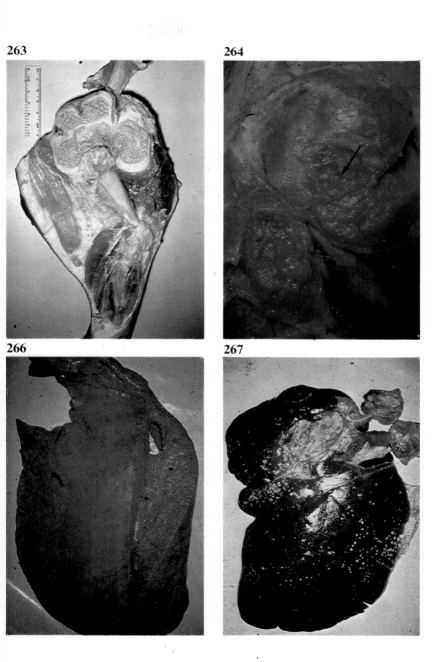

TUBERCULOSIS (BOVINE), cont.

268. HORSE SPLEEN. Miliary tuberculosis (**266–268** are from the same horse).

TUBERCULOSIS (SO CALLED SKIN TUBERCULOSIS)

269. BOVINE SUBCUTANEOUS TISSUE. The causal organism is a *Mycobacterium* of low pathogenicity. The lesions remain localised.

270. BOVINE SUBCUTANEOUS TISSUE.

TUMOURS

271. PIG OVARIES.

TYROSIN CRYSTALS

272. LAMB LIVERS. These are imported livers. Tyrosin, which is a normal constituent of liver, crystalises out. It is due to deterioration because of prolonged storage.

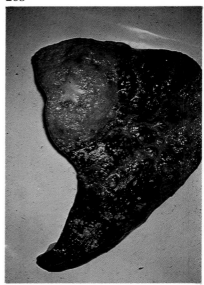

268

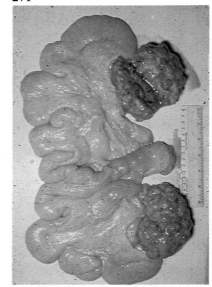

271

269

270

272

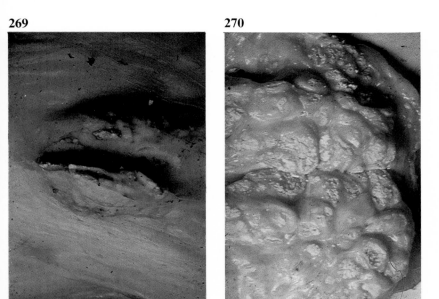

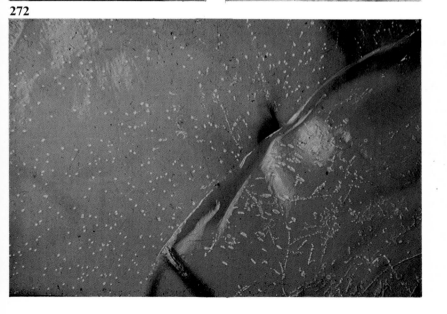

UMBILICAL PYAEMIA (OMPHALOPHLEBITIS)

273. CALF LIVER. The umbilical cord is very much enlarged and contains pus. There are numerous abscesses in the substance of the liver (see **11**).

UMBILICAL PYAEMIA, cont.

274. CALF LIVER (see **11**).

WARBLE FLY LARVA *(HYPODERMA BOVIS)*

275. BOVINE KIDNEY. The larva *(arrow)* wanders throughout the body and reaches the subcutaneous tissue of the back (as does *Hypoderma lineatum*, **276**).

WARBLE FLY LARVA *(HYPODERMA LINEATUM)*

276. BOVINE OESOPHAGUS. The larvae leave the oesophagus during January and February and travel towards the subcutaneous tissue of the back (see **277**).

WARBLE FLY LARVA ('LICKED' BACK OR 'LICKED' BEEF)

277. BOVINE SUBCUTANEOUS TISSUE OF THE BACK. This is the larva of *Hypoderma bovis* or *Hypoderma lineatus*. In spring the mature larva emerges from its cyst and falls to the ground, into which it burrows to pupate.

273

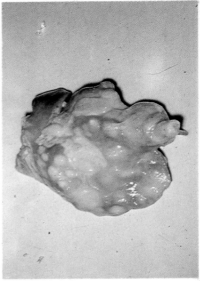

274

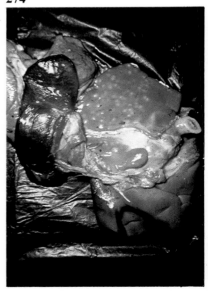

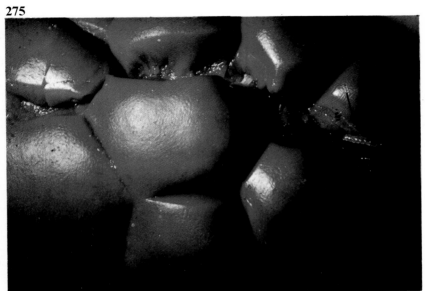

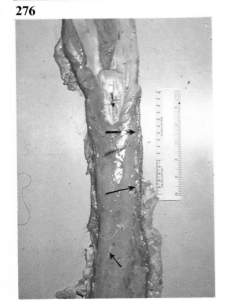

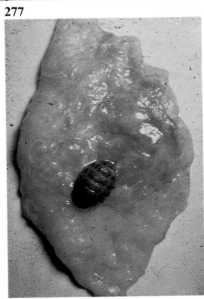

WHARTON'S JELLY

278. CALF LIVER. This is an accumulation of fluid which collects under the peritoneal covering of the liver.

WHITE HEIFER DISEASE

279. BOVINE UTERUS. Fluid accumulates in the uterus because of an imperforate hymen. This occurs in white heifers of the Shorthorn breed.

XANTHOSIS

280. BOVINE DIAPHRAGM AND ADRENAL GLAND. Normal diaphragm and adrenal glands are shown below for comparison. The cause is unknown.

281. BOVINE HEART. Shown with a normal heart.

282. BOVINE MUSCLE. Shown with a normal muscle.

YELLOW FATTED SHEEP

283. SHEEP. The yellow fatted sheep on the left is shown with a jaundiced sheep on the right.

278

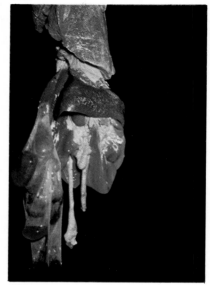

281

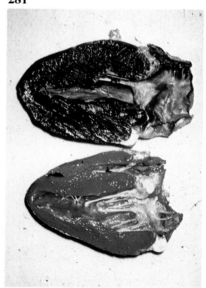

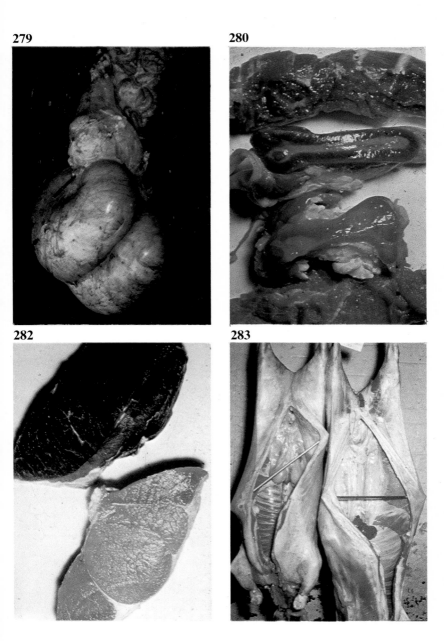

279

280

282

283

Poultry

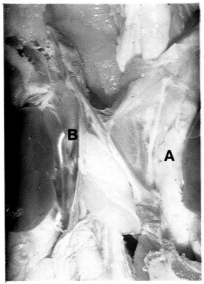

AIR SAC INFECTION

284. FOWL. The causal organism is *Mycoplasma gallisepticum.* Two fowl have been placed side by side to show an affected air sac in one (A) filled with pus, and a normal healthy air sac (B) in the other. The condition mainly affects young chickens.

ASCARIDIA GALLI

285. FOWL INTESTINE. Note how the intestine is completely blocked by worms. The photograph is of a bird which died.

285

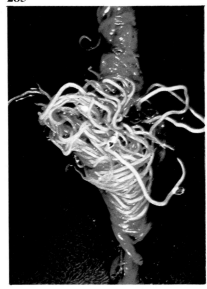

ASCITES

286. FOWL. Note the swollen abdomen indicating the excessive accumulation of fluid, which is easily diagnosed by palpation.

BLACKHEAD (INFECTIOUS ENTERO HEPATITIS. HISTOMONIASIS)

287. TURKEY LIVER. The causal organism is *Histomonas meleagridis.*

288. TURKEY LIVER. The lesions are more chronic than in **287**.

289. TURKEY INTESTINES. Note the impacted caeca (*arrows*).

BLACKSPOT MOULD

290. TURKEY. The causal organism is *Cladosporium herbarum.*

BLOOD SPLASHING

291. TURKEY. Note the haemorrhages in the breast muscles (A). Portions of breast muscle which have been roasted are shown at B. Note the colour change of haemorrhages from red to black.

286

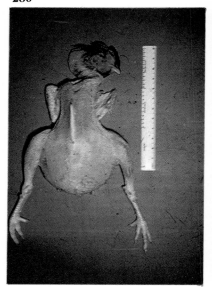

289

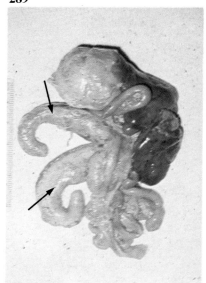

287

288

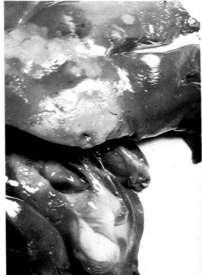

290

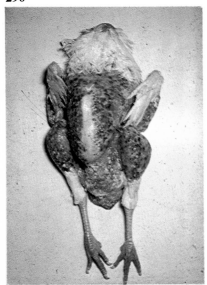

291

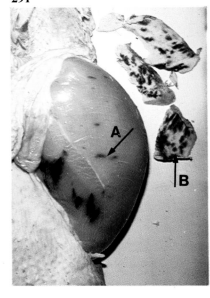

BREAST BLISTER ABSCESS
292. FOWL. This is caused by an injury to the skin and tissues over the sternum (*arrow*) which is often involved. The injury has become septic and an abscess has formed (see **337**).

BRUISING
293. FOWL.

BUMBLEFOOT
294. TURKEY. The cause is trauma or infection or both. The most common infection is by staphylococci.

CARCINOMA
295. FOWL. Note the cancerous ovary (*arrow*) and the large number of abnormal ova.

COCCIDIOSIS (CAECAL)
296. FOWL. The causal organism is *Eimeria tenella*. Note the bloodstained contents of the caeca.

COCCIDIOSIS (INTESTINAL)
297. FOWL. The causal organisms are *Eimeria necatrix* and *Eimeria acervulina*. Note the numerous haemorrhages in the small intestine (*arrow*).

292

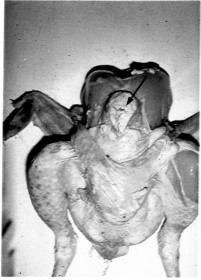

295

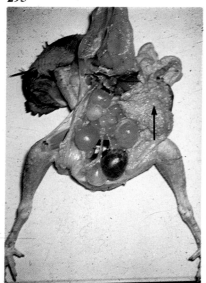

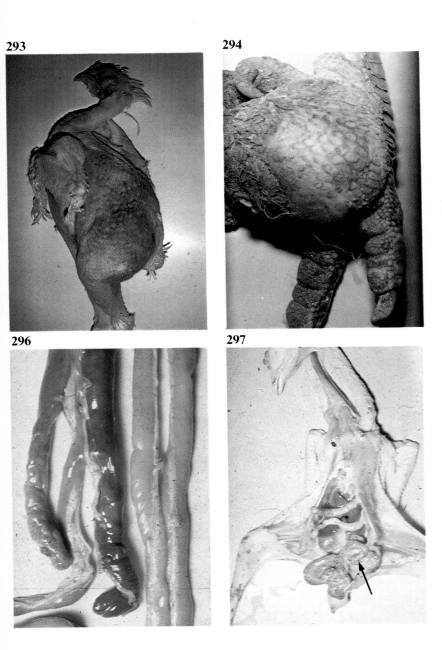

293

294

296

297

COLI GRANULOMA (HJÄRRE'S DISEASE)

298. FOWL INTESTINE. The causal organism is *Escherichia coli*. This follows an *E. coli* septicaemia. Compare with pustular typhilitis (**330**) and tuberculosis of the intestine (**340**). The specimen is from a bird that died.

CURLY TOE (CURLED TOE PARALYSIS)

299. FOWL. This is due to a deficiency of vitamin B_2.

EMPHYSEMA

300. FOWL. Note the subcutaneous emphysema due to a fracture of the humerus, which is hollow and connected to the air sacs. This has allowed air to infiltrate into the subcutaneous tissue.

E. COLI INFECTION

301. FOWL. The causal organism is *Esherichia coli*. This is in an acute stage showing inflammation and mottling of the liver.

E. COLI SEPTICAEMIA (see also figure 298)

302. FOWL. Chronic type in which the viscera, especially the liver, becomes covered with a fibrinous exudate. This generally follows a mycoplasma infection.

303. FOWL. Chronic type with fibrinous exudate and a layer of pus covering the liver.

298

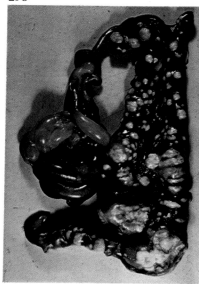

301

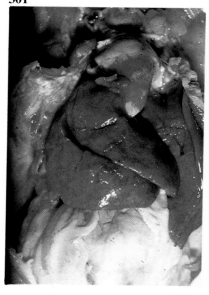

299

300

302

303

FIBROMA
304. FOWL. Note the large tumour (*arrow*).

305. FOWL PERITONEUM. Note the numerous tumours around the intestine.

FOREIGN BODIES
306. TURKEY GIZZARD. Note the two wire nails penetrating the gizzard and the toy bullet in the gizzard.

FOWL POX
307. FOWL. The causal organism is a virus. Note the typical lesions about the face. They may also appear on the legs, feet, under the wings and around the cloaca.

FOWL TYPHOID
308. FOWL. The causal organism is *Salmonella gallinarum*. Note the typical bronzed liver, abnormal ova and dark brown marrow.

FREEZER BURN
309. TURKEY. The burns are seen as white and dark patches. They are due to prolonged or over-refrigeration.

304

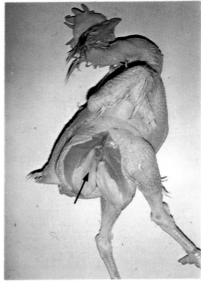

307

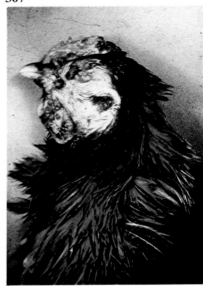

305

306

308

309

GAPES

310. FOWL TRACHEA. The causal organism is *Syngamus trachea*. The male and female worms are permanently attached in copulation. The males are very much smaller than the females.

GOUT

311. FOWL. One swelling has been incised to show the accumulation of salts of uric acid. There is also a visceral type of gout in which the salts are deposited on the surface of the heart, liver etc.

INFECTIVE SINUSITIS ('SWELL HEAD')

312. TURKEY. The causal organism is a mycoplasma.

313. TURKEY. The swelling has been opened to show the contained pus.

310

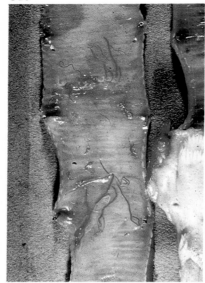

311

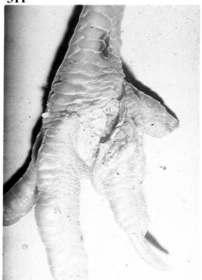

312

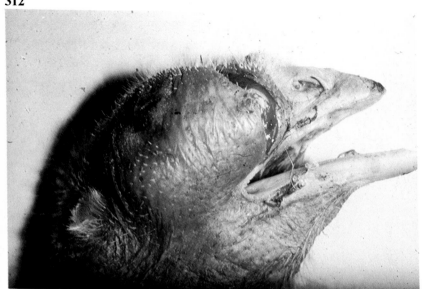

313

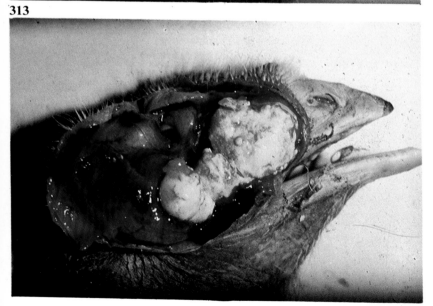

INFECTIVE SYNOVITIS

314. FOWL. The causal organism is *Mycoplasma synoviae.*

LYMPHOID LEUCOSIS (VISCERAL LYMPHOMATOSIS, BIG LIVER DISEASE)

315. FOWL. The causal organism is a virus. Note the very large, pale liver.

316. FOWL. Note the large liver and the numerous white tumours, especially affecting the heart. It is not possible to differentiate macroscopically these tumours from Marek's disease tumours.

317. FOWL LIVERS. Note the numerous tumours in the substance of the livers.

318. FOWL VISCERA. Note the tumours in the spleen (A) and kidney (B).

MANDIBULAR DISEASE ('SHOVEL BEAK')

319. FOWL. Note the distortion and necrosis of the lower mandibles, said to be due to excessively dry feeding.

314

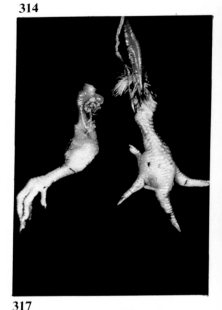

317

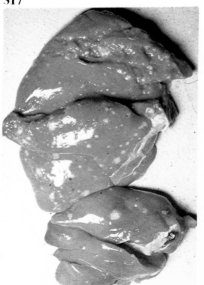

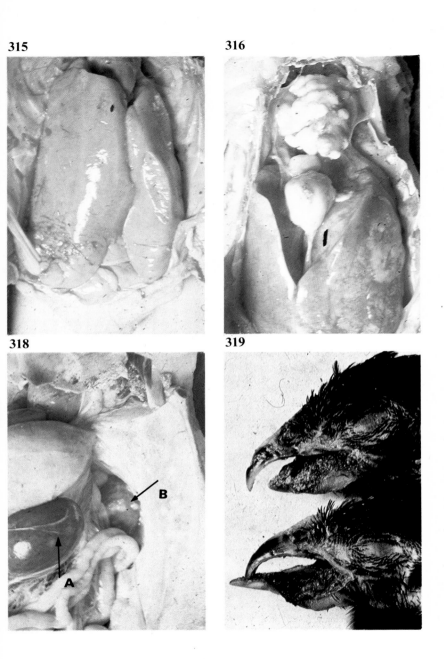

315

316

318

319

MAREK'S DISEASE

320. FOWL SKIN. The causal organism is a virus. The tumours appear as swellings (*arrow*).

321. FOWL LIVER. The tumours are similar to those of lymphoid leucosis but tend to be larger and more circumscribed.

322. FOWL LIVER.

MAREK'S DISEASE (NEURAL LYMPHOMATOSIS, FOWL PARALYSIS)

323. FOWL NERVE. Typical enlarged nerves of the sciatic plexus (A). Compare with normal nerves (B).

OREGON BREAST MUSCLE DISEASE (DEGENERATIVE MYOPATHY)

324. TURKEY. The disease is hereditary and the lesions are believed to be due to a failure of the blood supply to that part of the breast muscle called the fillet breast muscle. Depressions are seen (*arrows*) due to the loss of muscle tissue.

325. TURKEY. There is almost complete disappearance of the fillet part of the breast muscle exposing the sternum below (A). Compare with the normal turkey (B).

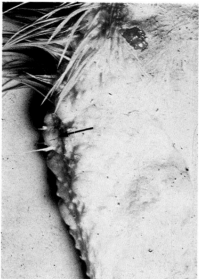

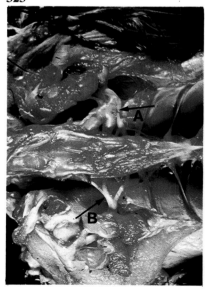

321

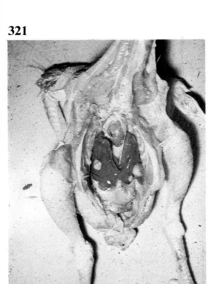

322

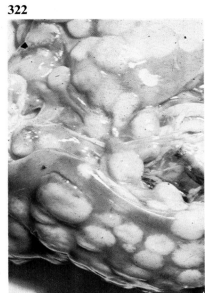

324

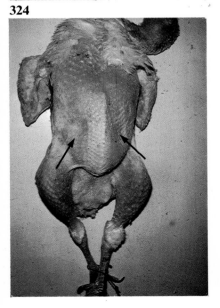

325

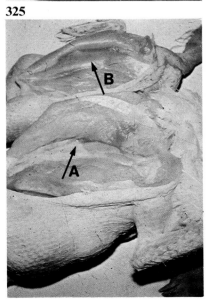

OREGON BREAST MUSCLE DISEASE, cont.

326. TURKEY. Note the abnormal colours resulting from the muscle degeneration (*arrows*).

OSTEOPETROSIS (PAGET'S DISEASE, THICK LEG DISEASE or MARBLE BONE)

327. FOWL. Gross thickening of the leg bones is apparent. Other bones may also be affected.

PEROSIS ('SLIPPED TENDON')

328. FOWL. This is due to a deficiency of manganese. The hock joints become deformed and the gastrocnemius tendons slip out of the grooves between the condyles. This causes the 'knock-kneed' appearance.

PLANTAR NECROSIS

329. FOWL. There is necrosis and exfoliation of the skin of the plantar surface of the foot (see **337**).

PUSTULAR TYPHILITIS

330. FOWL CAECA. The cause is unknown. This may be confused with coli granuloma (**298**) and tuberculosis of the intestine (**340**).

PUTREFACTION AND ASCITES

331. FOWL. The putrefaction is seen as the green colour (*arrow*). See figure **286**, ascites.

326

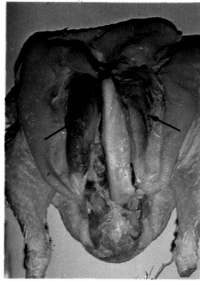

329

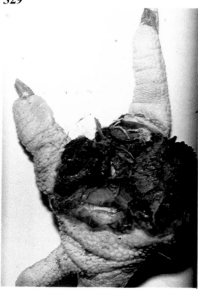

327

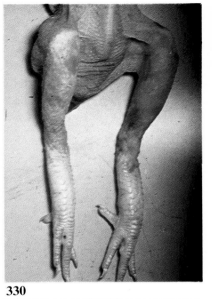

328

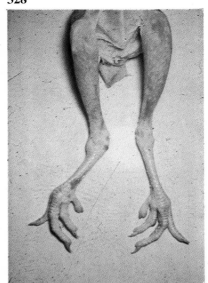

330

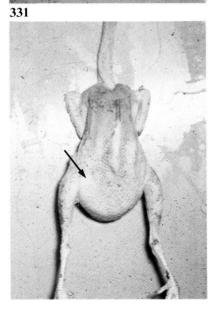

331

RICKETS
332. FOWL. The cause is a vitamin D deficiency. Enlargement of the bones is seen at A and B, bending of the bone at C. The keel of the sternum is twisted.

ROUND HEART DISEASE
333. TURKEY. The heart is ballooned and round (A) and the liver is enlarged with rounded borders (B). This is thought to be a metabolic disorder.

RUPTURED GASTRO-CNEMIUS TENDONS
334. FOWL. The cause is unknown. A normal fowl is shown for comparison.

RUPTURED OVIDUCT
335. FOWL. The partly formed eggs are lying in the abdomen. There is some doubt whether this is due to rupture of the oviduct or to reverse peristalsis in the oviduct.

SCALY LEG
336. FOWL. Caused by the scaly leg mite *Cnemidocoptes mutans*.

332

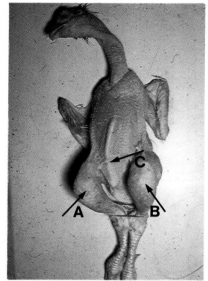

333

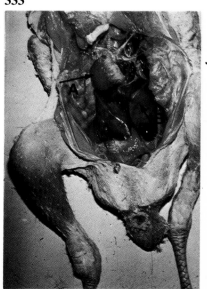

334

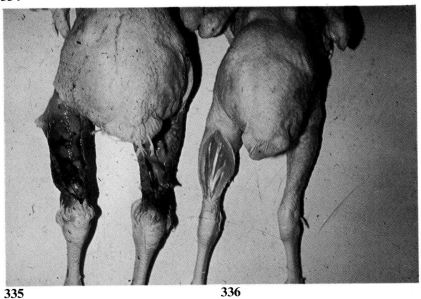

335

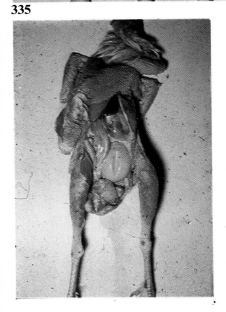

336

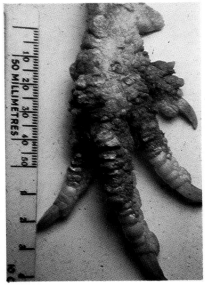

SORE HOCKS, BREAST BLISTER AND PLANTAR NECROSIS
337. FOWL. (See **292** and **329**.)

TISSUE MITE
338. FOWL. The mites, *Laminosioptes cysticola,* are encapsulated in the nodules just under the skin.

TUBERCULOSIS
339. FOWL. The causal organism is *Mycobacterium avium* (*M. tuberculosis,* avian strain). Compare the fowl on the left, suffering from tuberculosis emaciation, with the normal fowl on the right.

340. FOWL LUNG, INTESTINE AND STERNUM. Note the nodules in the lung (A), intestine (B) and sternum (C). Compare with coli granuloma (**298**) and pustular typhilitis (**330**).

341. FOWL LIVER, SPLEEN AND FEMUR. Note the nodules in the liver (A), spleen (B) and femur (C).

XANTHOMATOSIS
342. FOWL. The skin is thickened and yellow. The cause is unknown.

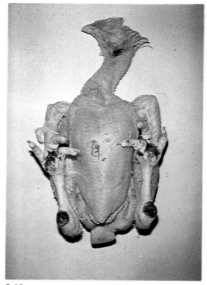

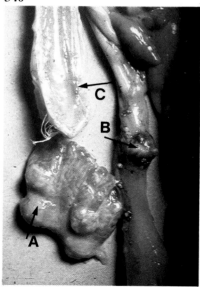

338

339

341

342

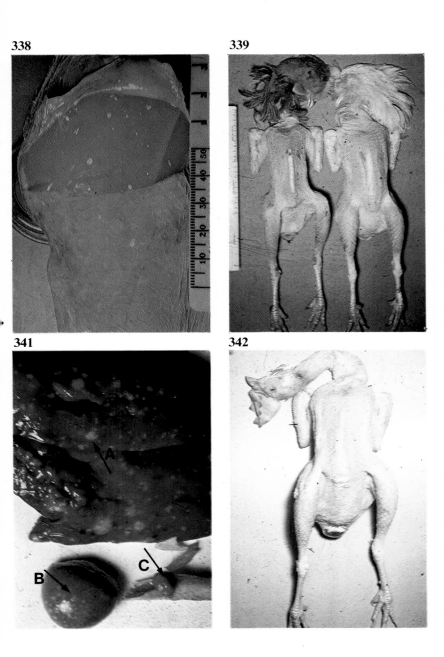

Index

Numbers refer to illustrations